Fasting and Autophagy for the Common Mann

Kelly Gregg MD

Published by Kelly Gregg, 2023.

FASTING AND AUTOPHAGY FOR THE COMMON MANN

First edition. September 26, 2023.

Copyright © 2023 Kelly Gregg MD.

ISBN: 979-8223342427

Written by Kelly Gregg MD.

FASTING AND AUTOPHAGY FOR THE COMMON MAN

Fasting and Autophagy for the Common Man

Kelly Gregg MD

209

CHAPTER 1
Fasting

This book continues the series of diet and health. In every book, I mention fasting, usually no more than one chapter. I am afraid I have given the impression that fasting is optional in the pursuit of good health. This has motivated me to write a little more extensively about this topic as now I believe it may be a necessary part of your diet to maintain good health.

Throughout my life, I have heard many diet recommendations. Most are general such as eat more vegetables or eat less sugar. I never heard the recommendation to fast more. In fact, I never heard the recommendation to fast at all. I have never heard a health care provider make a recommendation to anyone to fast to help lose weight, even though common sense would tell us that this must be the best way to reduce fat. Why is it that the medical field completely ignores this treatment?

I may have misspoken. It is modern medicine that has ignored this treatment. Fasting as a treatment has been practiced for thousands of years. In some of our oldest written documents in the western world, fasting is mentioned; both as a treatment for disease or an attempt to attain mental clarity.

Often. thousands of years ago, it was associated with a spiritual practice of some kind to attain some type of revelation or peace. I believe modern man ascribe this practice as the pursuit of some type of denial such that the man then felt he deserved some type of revelation. Somehow by not eating he was pleasing whatever God he worshipped. As my studies on diet have continued, I now believe the fasting state did not only psychologically prepare the mind, but physiologic changes in the brain as a result of fasting may have led to insight into various problems, or perhaps facilitated the communication between the conscious and unconscious mind.

The Greeks where big fans of observation of the natural world. They recognized that animals will often fast when they are ill. They also recognized that some diseases markedly decreased one's appetite. Throughout history, physicians (healers) in many different cultures have used fasting as a treatment. In the early 1900s, fasting became popular to treat various illnesses in the United States and Europe.

I have often noticed that modern society often discounts the knowledge gathered by mankind over thousands of years, supposing these individuals were primitive whose thinking could be discounted. Do you believe man is smarter now than 3000 years ago? Just because you know how to operate a cell phone does not mean you could survive in the woods. You may know how to operate a computer, but could you build one? Could you even make the plastic cover? Could you even make an iron nail? Fasting was used throughout history because it provided some type of beneficial effect. Man was smart enough to abandon it if it did not work and, in many cultures, or historical eras, fasting was practiced.

At this point I need to clarify the definition of fasting. Fasting for our purposes, meaning in the context of diet and health, means no caloric intake. I will count the consumption of a substance with less than one calorie (such as coffee) as being zero. Vitamins may be taken as well as electrolytes (bone broth). It is important to note that fasting is not starvation as long as you have fat stores for energy. I am interested in maintaining health and we should not have to worry about any complications.

To understand what happens when we are fasting, we will have to understand what happens when we eat. This will require a little biochemistry, nothing you will not readily understand simply using your common sense. Then we can progress to what happens when you do not eat.

In almost all my diet and health books, I must include these chapters. In almost all my books, I will also refer to the Angus fast, one that lasted 382 days. I will discuss fasting more extensively in this book and include additional information about the subject. I will tell you upfront that as a minimum, you must maintain twelve hours of fasting between your last intake of calories in the day, to your first intake of calories the next day. This should be no big deal and you probably do this almost all the time now.

To understand the role of fasting in diet and health, you must understand autophagy. I will explain this homeostatic mechanism in this book. It will make sense to you.

My current books which are part of a tetralogy are:

Diabetes, Prediabetes, Obesity management, prevention, treatment

The Ketogenic Diet for Beginners
Fasting and Autophagy for the Common Man
Maintenance Diet for the Modern Man
Bread in the Modern Diet

These all stand separately as people have different needs. At the same time, if you wanted to buy all of them separately, it would be too expensive, and the information would overlap. As such, all these books are combined into one in the book *DIET AND HEALTH*. Right now, we are interested in fasting, and the first part of this book will give you the information you need.

Now the disclaimer. Do not consider anything I say to you to be medical advice. I am a retired physician and no longer in practice. That does not mean what I say is not good advice.

CHAPTER 2
Food

I cannot really communicate with you unless we all start with some basic information. Like most science, the difficulty is in learning the language. Almost everyone has enough common sense to figure it out if we agree on the basic terms. That is why it seems like every book I write must include this chapter and possibly the next, so if you have read any of my books, you may have already read something like this.

I originally did not want to cut and paste this portion of the book from my other books, but there are only so many ways to say the same thing. Also, I have continuously refined the information so that I think it now is rather good and difficult for me to improve upon. Therefore, you may feel cheated if you have read some of my other books. Of course, if you have read them, you probably do not need to read this chapter anyway. If you only know the basics of nutrition, say the metabolic equivalent of long division, you need to read it. If you know the metabolic equivalent of calculus, just read the first and last sentence of every paragraph. If you know the metabolic equivalent of solving quantum wave equations, skip this chapter.

Your food is divided up into fats, carbohydrates, and protein. About 99% of what you eat goes into one of these categories. In this book, I am not going to care about vitamins and minerals. It is rare in this country that anyone suffers from a real vitamin deficiency disease such as rickets or scurvy. In the United States, in one day we probably urinate out enough vitamins to satisfy the requirements of the rest of the world for a week. Someday I will write about vitamins, but then I will have to go into witness protection from everyone getting mad at me.

Let's start with fats. Fats come in two basic forms. One is a chain of carbon atoms of varying lengths which are termed a fatty acid. These usually have between 4 and 28 carbon atoms. Sometimes these carbon atoms are linked together in what is called a double bond. Saturated fatty acids mean no double bonds, unsaturated means one or more double bonds. Saturated fatty acids are more likely to be solid at normal temperatures, unsaturated more likely to be liquid. When someone says something like omega 3 fatty acid, that means the first double bond is at the third carbon from the omega end. An omega 6 fatty acid means double at the 6 carbon. The omega end is the end opposite the COOH (Carboxyl) group.

There is a lot of misunderstanding among both professionals and laypeople about the role of saturated versus unsaturated fatty acids My view; saturated fats are not bad for you.

For the most part, that is all the biochemistry you need to know. You will hear these terms used and now at least you kind of know what they are talking about. In real life, you do not eat fatty acids. You take three fatty acids, hook them up to a glycerol molecule, and you get a triglyceride. This is what you are eating with a piece of bacon. It is a much more compact way to store fat and does not use up as many water molecules, so this is the way nature works. When you eat fat, your stomach acids and digestive enzymes break down the triglycerides into component fatty acids, which can be different in the same triglyceride. This is what is absorbed into the body, not the triglyceride. Unlike carbohydrates and proteins, most fatty acids are absorbed through the lymphatic system and dumped into the bloodstream.

The other foods are absorbed and pumped right to the liver before entering the blood. That way the liver gets the first crack at the food and whatever else you may have eaten. If it was something bad for you, the liver gets a chance to neutralize it before it goes to the rest of the body. Sometimes it doesn't get to it on the first pass, but the liver gets more chances as the blood circulates. We divide the triglycerides up into short-chain triglycerides that have less than six carbons in the fatty acids, medium-chain with six to twelve carbons, and long-chain with twelve or more carbons. This means that at least two out of the three fatty acids in the triglyceride have this length. Yes, a triglyceride does not have to have three identical fatty acids. The medium-chain fatty acids (like in coconut oil) can get absorbed directly into the bloodstream and skip the lymphatic system; hence, they can more rapidly be used by the body for fuel.

To sum it up, we eat fats, and your wonderful digestive system breaks them down into fatty acids in the gut. These fatty acids are then absorbed in the small intestine and converted back into triglycerides. Many of these triglycerides are then converted into chylomicrons. These are particles containing triglycerides and apolipoproteins (which allow them to remain in solution) and transported in the lymphatic system to the subclavian vein (at the junction of your neck and shoulder) where they are dumped into the blood. I will talk about apolipoproteins later in the book.

These triglycerides are then used by the liver and other cells. This trip from the lymphatic system to the blood takes a while. Meanwhile, the medium-chain triglycerides are converted into fatty acids and are absorbed and bound to albumin instead of forming chylomicrons. These enter the portal vein and go directly to the liver, skipping the lymphatic system. They are then processed or dumped into the blood for energy usage. As you can see, medium-chain fatty acids are treated differently as they go directly to the liver. It takes a lot longer to travel through the lymphatic system than just through the portal vein.

Fatty acids are used in the body for energy. Most of the energy use in the body is just to keep you alive and warm. Exercise, by which I mean, just walking around and doing normal stuff, only accounts for about 20% of your energy use; the rest is the brain and other organs. Your body is very stingy about energy. Once it gets some through eating, which is the only way your body gets energy, it wants to keep it. So, if you eat fat, it gets turned into fatty acids, and eventually into the bloodstream (in the form of both fatty acids and triglycerides). Your body does not want to waste it. Some is absorbed by the cells and used right away for energy, but the rest is stored to be used later.

You already know that these fatty acids are stored in your fat cells. Fatty acids are absorbed by the fat cells and can be converted into triglyceride which is the form of fat stored in your fat cells. Your fat cells can also go the other direction and turn triglycerides into fatty acids, which are then secreted to the blood. We will see later that perhaps the main source of this fat in the fat cells comes from glucose, not fatty acids.

I'll bet you can figure out what hormone controls which way the fat cell is going: making fat or breaking down triglycerides. Yep, it's insulin. High insulin makes the fat cell want to take up fatty acids and glucose; low insulin levels make the fat cell want to secrete fatty acids. The hormone glucagon may actually be the main driver of fatty acid release, but that only goes up if insulin goes down. The fatty acids conveniently released by the fat cells to be used as energy are carried by albumin, the proteins in the liquid part of the blood; as you can imagine, fat does not dissolve in water very well.

I must interject an additional message about fat. Much of the fat that ends up in the blood, in the form of triglycerides carried by lipoproteins like LDL, comes not from the diet, but are derived from the production of fat from fructose and glucose by the liver. In other words, if you had low fat intake, but lots of carbohydrates, you would still get lipoproteins in the blood. Both the liver and the fat cells are in the business of making fat from sugar.

Next on the list is protein. You probably know what protein is. It is meat. You know what it looks like and that we normally cook it. You already know your muscles are composed of protein. But wait a minute, what about those vegetarians. Well, plants contain plenty of protein. It does not look exactly like animal protein (although soy burgers are close), but it gets turned into muscle just like pork chops do. Proteins are made of amino acids. There are about 20 different amino acids we use to build everything in the body. Proteins are often large molecules containing hundreds of amino acids. All your enzymes are proteins.

Your hormones sometimes contain protein. Your heart, lungs, liver, kidneys, and skin are mainly protein. Of course, don't forget those pecs. There are eight or nine essential amino acids: These are amino acids we cannot make ourselves and must acquire through diet. We can make the rest.

Proteins are usually broken down into their component amino acids and absorbed by the gut to be used by the body to make things. Sometimes they are not completely broken down and actual proteins can get absorbed, which sometimes causes a problem with the immune system. We need about 2-3 ounces of protein a day, but often eat a lot more. The extra can be used for energy and can be converted into glucose.

Now the main event: carbohydrates. Carbohydrates are sugar molecules. Diabetes is elevated sugar in the blood, and by that, I mean glucose. Insulin controls glucose in that it enhances the absorption of glucose into various cells in the body. We already know about type one diabetes mellitus (T1DM), that it is a defect in the production of insulin in young people, probably secondary to the autoimmune destruction of the cells that make insulin. Now we are going to talk about Type 2 Diabetes, T2DM, which is also elevated blood sugar; but we arrive there by a different pathway. Eventually, many with T2DM end up in the same place as T1DM; not enough insulin to control blood sugar. We need to understand that elevated blood glucose can be directly harmful to many cells and organs in the body. It also contributes to advanced glycation end products, something I will explain later.

Your body does not like very low insulin like type 1 diabetes, or very high insulin. It does not like very low blood sugar like hypoglycemia, or very high blood sugar. We need to see how sugar is metabolized in the body and how insulin reacts to sugar in the body to understand diabetes. It is also important to understand that insulin resistance is going to be the basis for T2DM.

A single sugar molecule is called a monosaccharide. There are three main monosaccharides and glucose is the primary one. Some fruits contain free glucose, and honey is about one-third glucose and one-third fructose, but usually, glucose is combined another sugar molecule: often another glucose. The important sugar monosaccharide sugar molecules are glucose, fructose, and galactose.

There are also three main disaccharides: that is sugars that contain two sugar molecules. These are sucrose, lactose, and maltose. I have found confusion reigns in this area so let's try to straighten things out.

Sucrose is table sugar. This is a combination of glucose and fructose. Your body easily splits these two apart and absorbs them rapidly. Remember, glucose is the only sugar to which your pancreas responds with the secretion of insulin. Your pancreas is usually quite good at this and can secrete lots of insulin.

Fructose is found in fruits. This is the only single sugar (monosaccharide) of any importance in the diet. In fruit it is combined with fiber, hence it takes your gut awhile to get it absorbed, as opposed to table sugar which is rapidly split into fructose and glucose and rapidly taken up.

Lactose is a combination of glucose and galactose, and often found in dairy products and milk. This is of importance in that some individuals lose the activity of the enzyme to split these two sugars apart as they get older and cannot digest lactose. The bacteria in the colon sure can and this leads to the production of gas and bowel discomfort. Other than this, lactose is not too important in adults. The galactose and glucose are absorbed, and the galactose converted into glucose.

Maltose is simply two glucose molecules. Starch in plants is composed of long chains of glucose molecules. Your digestive tract splits off two molecules of glucose at a time which is maltose. Then it splits the maltose into individual glucose molecules which are absorbed in the usual way. In the typical American diet, we get most of our calories from starches in the form of wheat and potatoes. Just think, hamburger buns and French fries are mainly starch, which is saying they are mainly sugar, and that sugar is mainly glucose.

Starches are long chains of glucose molecules, as is cellulose. In cellulose (wood) these glucose molecules are bound together differently from starches, and we do not have the enzyme to break them apart: hence they are not digested or absorbed. This is why when you look at the label on food and it lists the total carbohydrate content in grams, it divides the carbohydrates into sugar and fiber. If you are counting carbs, you get to subtract the grams of fiber from the total carbs.

Some animals can break apart the glucose bonds in cellulose and use the resulting glucose for energy or convert it into fat. I know, it's really the bacteria in their stomachs that break it apart. It turns out that the bacteria in our colon can break down this fiber somewhat resulting in components that can be used for energy by our colon cells. It can also result in fatty acid production and volatile gases, which have been demonstrated by generations of teenage boys to be flammable.

A quick review of sugars shows you that the main driver of energy in the human body is going to be glucose. Most of the cells of the human body can use glucose to produce energy to keep you alive. Insulin facilitates the uptake of glucose by the cells of the body; however, your brain is so important it does not need insulin to use glucose. Throughout recorded history, carbohydrates have been the main source of energy for the human body. One of the reasons is that it can be preserved easily to use in times of decreased food supply. It didn't take our ancestors long to figure this out. You can't store a leg of lamb very long, but you can put whole wheat kernels in a sealed clay pot and store them for years.

CHAPTER 3
Eating

Now that we know what food is, back to what happens when we eat. In order to understand what happens when we don't eat, we must know what happens when we do. We are concerned with carbohydrates, mainly glucose and fructose, whether in table sugar, fruit, or starch. Later I will talk a little about high fructose corn syrup. It won't be good.

Put food in your mouth. The first thing that happens is that you taste the food. If it tastes terrible you spit it out, which for the most part is a good thing. Terrible tasting food is usually not good for you as it may be poison. Don't be afraid to spit something out. The taste of food occurs in the brain and is tied to our psychology. Sweet taste is desirable to the brain. That makes sense since the brain likes glucose. Bitter is a slight warning, but a little is OK, sour again a slight warning. Salty is something we can desire under certain circumstances. Umami is a meat-like taste that may drive us to protein. Taste is complex and another book. For our glucose attention, saliva contains an enzyme that can cleave starch into maltose molecules in the mouth. Remember maltose is two glucose molecules. This is not as sweet as fructose.

There exists a cephalic phase of insulin secretion which occurs even before any glucose hits the gut. Although this is not large, it does occur before you start eating. It also occurs when you think about food or when you see an ad on TV about pizza or donuts. As you may realize, eating multiple times a day results in multiple episodes of insulin secretion, regardless of the blood sugar. The basic pathophysiology of T2DM and obesity may revolve around insulin resistance. As you get multiple surges of insulin daily, and these surges occur more often, are of a higher peak, and occur more rapidly, you may slowly desensitize your insulin receptors to insulin. You may be inducing your body to make fewer insulin receptors, as there always seems to be plenty of insulin around so we can save energy by not making as many. Eventually, you need a little more to get the same effect. Now we have insulin level creep, as well as baseline glucose level creep. After 20-30 years, we now have obesity and prediabetes.

The stomach then sterilizes the food and begins the digestion of fat and protein. Carbos finally reach small intestines. Most of the time glucose is tied up in sucrose and starch. Sucrose is rapidly divided into glucose and fructose which are then rapidly absorbed by different mechanisms. Glucose goes into the blood then directly to the liver which then sends it to the bloodstream. The glucose is detected by the pancreas and here comes the insulin.

Back to the liver. The liver also stores glycogen. Glycogen is like animal starch. It is a highly branched string of glucose molecules the liver can break apart one glucose molecule at a time. The liver makes sure the brain is happy by keeping the glucose level stable by either releasing glucose from glycogen or making glucose out of protein. Remember you have lots of protein, even more than fat. The liver is always adding or subtracting from its glycogen supply.

Your body is stingy about glucose. Once the plasma glucose level gets around 200 mg/dl, glucose begins to be lost in the urine. Your body does not like that, so it tries to save glucose energy. It does this by secreting insulin which hastens the absorption of glucose by the cells of the body, especially the muscle cells. The higher the plasma sugar, the more insulin is secreted. It also tries to save energy by storing it in fat cells. Glucose goes into the fat cell, is converted to fatty acids, and then saved as triglycerides. The higher the insulin, the more this process takes place. If you happen to have low insulin, this process goes in the other direction; however, once the glucose is converted to fatty acids by the fat cells, it does not go back to glucose. Fatty acids are released instead.

High levels of glucose are directly toxic to cells in the body, so if it gets too high, getting rid of it in the urine is the last resort. Chronically high glucose may be a factor in the ultimate destruction of the beta insulin-producing cells in the pancreas and result in low insulin levels in T2DM. Your body is going to keep absorbing it as long as you keep eating it. For every glucose molecule in table sugar, there is a fructose molecule (the two molecules together make one sucrose molecule). Fructose does not stimulate insulin production and insulin does not enhance the absorption of fructose by the cells. Virtually all metabolism of fructose takes place in the liver. A little is used by the sperm for energy. When it hits the liver, it is used to make glycogen. The leftover is converted into fatty acids and triglycerides. It takes a while for the liver to do this, so the fructose wanders around in your bloodstream a while. Later I'll tell you why you don't want this.

So, let's be clear. You eat sucrose (table sugar) and get glucose and just as much fructose. The glucose gets gobbled up by the tissue to be used as energy. The fructose gets turned into glucose and made into glycogen by the liver, it also turns a lot of the fructose into fatty acids and hence to triglycerides, just like the fat cells. These triglycerides are not saved in the liver(although it does seem to contribute to fatty liver) but sent into blood bonded to what are called lipoproteins, which then carry them around to be used or saved in the fat cells along with the glucose derived triglyceride. Lipoproteins also carry cholesterol, a type of fat that is a sterol, that is not used directly for energy. To sum it up, glucose used directly for energy, fructose converted to glycogen (a string of glucose molecules) and the leftover converted into fatty acids/triglycerides. Fructose absorbed one to one with glucose, excess fructose and glucose may pass down the GI tract and eventually affect the gut microbiome.

The brain has a strange relationship with fructose. It does not absorb fructose to use it for energy. Recently we figured out that when your glucose levels get too high, the brain converts glucose into fructose. Remember a couple of things. Your brain does not need insulin to absorb glucose; hence controlling the insulin does not control the absorption. Elevated glucose levels are toxic to cells; even brain cells (maybe especially brain cells). If your glucose levels are elevated, lowering the insulin level does not keep the brain from absorbing it. The brain may be protecting itself from the elevated glucose levels by converting some of it to fructose. You don't want a lot of fructose floating around in your brain either. We will talk about Advanced Glycogen End Products (AGEs) later. Right now, you need to know you don't want a lot of them.

What is normal? That can change throughout your life. There is a metabolic and glucose setpoint in your body. Most people do not pay much attention to how much or what they eat. They eat when they are hungry and stop when they are full. Amazingly enough, this works pretty well. Most can keep their weight within a few pounds for years with little effort. As time goes on, we may notice a pound or two of weight gain a year. If our life changes dramatically the weight gain or loss may change more rapidly. But usually, we are minding our own business and suddenly realize after twenty or thirty years, that none of our clothes fit. Apparently, our set point has changed without our noticing it.

What changes that setpoint is more complicated and is related to age, activity, health, diet, and psychology. It does not matter. What we do know is that as your fasting glucose level slowly rises, your setpoint has risen.

Life is not fair, and some people eat a poor diet, get fat, don't exercise, and don't get T2DM. Like almost everything in life, your genes are going to be a major factor in what happens. What we do know is that obesity and T2DM have risen quite a bit in the last 150 years as compared to the previous 5000. Some may say it is just because we have more food. Some say it is because it is the type of food or the lack of exercise or that our genes have changed or maybe our gut biome is screwed up. No matter. We are looking for a diet that may prevent some of these modern diseases from occurring. We are not treating them, and if you have obesity or diabetes, you need one of my previous books. You then will need a different diet, not necessarily the diet for the modern man.

Your setpoint for the glucose level may change as you age. I mean like in 20 – 30 years. I am a little more confident that this is related to your diet. In most people, the problem isn't the pancreas not putting out enough insulin, it's the opposite. It's just the insulin isn't having the same effect. There is nothing wrong with the insulin, but rather the receptors on the cells don't seem to be using it as well. Let's give two examples that we already know about.

Your body changes as time goes on, your diet changes, or your activities change. If you start lifting weights, you may develop more lean body mass (muscles). You expect that to happen. You have induced certain biochemical processes in the muscle cells to use energy more efficiently or grow and repair more rapidly or operate better despite a lower oxygen supply or just look better. You did this by inducing certain metabolic processes that required enzymes or transport proteins. In other words, the DNA in the cells started replicating and producing RNA that coded for more proteins that cause increased absorption of amino acids that cause the ribosomes to make more molecules of various enzymes or receptors, that caused, well lots of things.

This does not happen overnight. It may take years to induce this activity to its full effect. The same can happen in reverse if you stop lifting weights. This induction of processes happens all over the body: Sometimes a little faster in certain cells, sometimes very slowly in certain cells.

Your skeletal muscle cells also have receptors for insulin on the surface of the cell. When stimulated by insulin it activates the process to absorb glucose (and by the way also amino acids) into the cell thus lowering the amount of glucose in the blood. The amount of glucose in the blood varies. If you are someone eating a lot of glucose, you will secrete more insulin. If you eat often, you will have more episodes of insulin secretion. Do this for 30 years. Over that time your muscle cells did not have to work that hard-to-get glucose. There was always plenty around at a high level and the cell did not have to work that hard to get it. Do you think that maybe you would induce the cell not to make as many insulin receptors?

Your body is fabulous. It will not waste energy making a lot of insulin receptors if it does not need a lot of receptors to get insulin. Over the years we know what happens. You need fewer receptors to get the job done. If we were always low on glucose, your body would make more receptors to suck out the glucose as fast as it can. High levels of glucose give lower numbers of receptors and no hurry to get the glucose sucked out, there is always plenty around.

Of course, your pancreas is not quite as smart, so it keeps pumping out a little more insulin to get that glucose down as it does not seem to be dropping as fast as it used to. Besides, the glucose receptors in the pancreas are always being exposed to a high level of glucose so they are not quite as sensitive to the blood level. The setpoint of the glucose level begins creeping up. After a while, you figure out what we get. The resting glucose level has gone up; however, the insulin level has also gone up. Eventually, we get what is called insulin resistance. Despite plenty of good insulin around, the blood level of glucose is higher.

In the meantime, let's see what those fat cells have been doing all these years. Insulin stimulates the fat cells to take up glucose and store it as fat. After all, the insulin levels would not be elevated unless the glucose level was elevated, and we want to save that energy. Similarly, if the insulin levels are low, that means the glucose level is low, and now we need to pump out fatty acids to give the body enough energy. The fat cells just care about insulin levels. In Type 1 diabetes, there is not enough insulin despite high glucose levels; hence the fat cells are not storing glucose. You get skinny children with high glucose levels.

If we have high insulin levels, guess what we are inducing. It is complicated to convert glucose into triglycerides and requires lots of different proteins and enzymes. If you have chronically elevated insulin levels, your fat DNA finally produces enough biochemical infrastructures that you get rather good at changing glucose into fat. This takes years to finally get up to speed, but once there it works great. At the same time, you have not been going the other way that often. You have not induced the conversion of triglycerides to fatty acids, so your fat stores are slowly getting bigger and bigger as if we hadn't already noticed that.

There is some hope. It's not quite as complicated to convert triglycerides to fat and does not take quite as long to induce. Although this process may not have been used for a while, it is more important to get energy out when needed than to add to an already large supply of stores. Hence your body is smart enough that this process can be induced faster if needed.

CHAPTER 4
<u>Not Eating</u>

Believe it or not, most of the time we are not eating. Everyone is familiar with getting a fasting blood test which most of the time means nothing to eat in the previous 12 hours. Sometimes we go longer than that without eating. Sometimes we go for one or two days, sometimes a month. What happens when we are not eating is important for us to understand.

We need energy to live. We can say that expending energy is life. The whole purpose of your body is to get energy. We only get energy through eating (there may be a tiny bit we get from sunshine but disregard that). Your body does a great job converting food to energy, using that energy, and saving enough so you do not usually run out. Your brain needs energy to think. You don't want to stop thinking because then you will stop working and no further food will be coming in. Your brain likes to use glucose. If you stop eating, you can see that perhaps slowly your glucose level will start dropping. After all, no glucose is coming in. Fatty acids may be released from fat cells but that is not glucose, and your brain does not use fatty acid for energy. Your fat cells can change glucose into fat but can't go the other direction. So how do we get those fasting blood tests and remain conscious?

Fortunately, your body is designed just for this circumstance. Remember that glycogen we stored in the liver. It contains about 100 grams of glucose and the liver breaks apart this large molecule of glucose units to keep the blood sugar from dropping too low and thus keeps your brain happy. It turns out that there are about 400 grams of glycogen in the muscle cells of the body, so despite not eating, you can still engage in vigorous exercise. This glycogen cannot be released into the circulation so it does not help the brain, but the muscles can keep functioning fine. Now, this does not last forever. After about one day you have used up the glycogen in the liver and muscles. What now?

When the insulin level drops, your liver in all its wisdom begins making its own glucose from protein. You have lots of protein and the liver is very good at making glucose. You could eat nothing for a month and your body would still have glucose floating around in the bloodstream. Of course, it takes a few hours for this process to get ginned up, and in the meantime, the low insulin level has stimulated glucagon to be released from the alpha cells in the pancreas.

Insulin comes from the beta cells. As insulin drops, glucagon goes up. One of the effects of glucagon is to get the fat cells to stop using up any glucose, we are going to save that for the brain, and start turning those triglycerides stored as fat into fatty acids and release these into the blood where they are carried around by albumin (the protein in the blood) and delivered throughout your body to be used as energy in place of glucose. Your liver is the star, but your kidneys also can make sugar from protein.

If you recall, a triglyceride is composed of three fatty acids bound to a glycerol molecule. This glycerol molecule can be taken up by the liver and used to make glucose just like the protein. Another effect of glucagon is to stimulate the release of epinephrine (adrenalin) which stimulates the muscles to break down glycogen and use that energy instead of sucking glucose out of the blood (again we are saving that for the brain).

Once we get the fatty acids in the blood, we have plenty of energy; in fact, fatty acids supply more energy per molecule than glucose. We still have this brain problem. There is a race between the liver making glucose, and the glycogen being depleted. Although the rest of your body is perfectly happy using fatty acids instead of glucose, your brain does not use fatty acids for energy. Whoever designed the liver knew what they were doing. As the fatty acids increase in the blood (and the glucose decreases), the liver begins making and releasing what are called ketone bodies into the blood. These are also left over from making new glucose. The primary ketone body is beta-hydroxybutyrate. These can be readily used by the brain for energy and to make long-chain fatty acids. There is some confusion as to whether the brain may even prefer to use ketone bodies for energy, but regardless, it remains happy if plenty of ketone bodies are around.

If we stop eating, numerous compensatory mechanisms kick in so that it is a rare event (unless medication is involved) that we pass out due to low blood sugar. Later I will talk about someone who did not eat carbohydrates for a year and never passed out.

There are various metabolic states in which your body exists, all are distinct. So far, we have eating, and not eating. There is a fasting metabolic state which is different from these.

There is also a feasting state (that enables you to eat that pecan pie at Thanksgiving even though you are completely stuffed), and a reduced-calorie metabolic state, which is why the reduced-calorie diet hardly ever works. These are different biochemical states. Your metabolic state is constantly changing in your body, and it's supposed to. The maintenance diet will hopefully keep you out of the reduced-calorie state. The 12 hours fast will at least start you in the fasting state. Don't eat for 24 hours and we are getting a good start on the fasting state.

CHAPTER 5
Metabolic States

I have given you a brief outline as to what happens between meals, and why your brain does not stop working a few hours after your last meal. I am now going to go into a little more detail about what happens when you stop taking in calories for a while, like for a week or two.

Let's agree on the definitions. Your body has numerous metabolic states and is transitioning between them all the time:

Starvation is a distinct metabolic state. It occurs when your body cannot generate energy from either fats or carbohydrates. Starvation is not feeling hungry. Although those in a starvation state do usually feel hungry, everyone who is hungry is not starving. It is rare in the US that we will find people starving. In starvation, your body is willing to metabolize all parts of the body to get energy. It is not a healthy state.

Fasting is not taking in calories. You drink whatever you want, but no calories (or less than one.) You will not really be in fasting state until you have had no caloric intake for 36 hours. The fasting state can be subdivided into a few metabolic states as your metabolism changes somewhat as the fast goes on. If you take in any calories, you are not in a fasting state but rather a reduced-calorie state.

A reduced-calorie state is one in which you are taking in fewer calories than your body is demanding to make energy. It is completely different from fasting and your body's reactions are different. Intermittent fasting has become popular, but you must take in no calories to get the benefits of fasting. I have already advised you that the reduced calorie diet is quite poor for weight loss. That is not to say that that fasting for 36 hours once or twice a week does not reap benefits, but it is not particularly a weight loss diet.

A ketogenic state is one in which few carbohydrates are taken in such that the body is using fat for energy, which results in ketones which show up in the urine. Although this is like what happens in fasting, it is a different metabolic state, and taking in calories, even though there are few carbs, does not give you the benefits of fasting. It turns out that this is a good fat loss diet, but eventually, you must go on a maintenance diet.

Back to fasting. We know that after a few hours the decreased insulin stimulates glucagon and the fat cells begin releasing fatty acids into the blood to provide energy. High insulin levels also usually suppress the production of glucose from the liver. Remember, there is always a little glucose being made by the liver, and one of the regulators of this production is insulin. As insulin drops, new glucose production increases.

The glucose produced by the metabolism of glycogen in the liver only lasts a day or so. The glycogen in the muscles also lasts about that long (depending on activity), and this glycogen cannot be released into the blood. It turns out the metabolites of the usage of this glycogen (lactate) can be released in the blood and the liver is happy to turn this into glucose.

The rate the liver and kidney make new glucose increases steadily for about a week, then falls off to a slightly lower rate, although much higher than it was when we were taking in carbs in our diet. Now all our glucose is homemade, but most of our energy is coming from fatty acids, so the glucose requirements for the body are much less. Within a few days, our blood glucose drops and stabilizes at a new, lower level.

This is all enabled by our breaking down the fat in the body, and, hence producing ketones. We are always converting glucose to fat in the fat cells. This rate is high with high glucose. We also convert fat to fatty acids all the time. This rate is high with low glucose. As we start fasting, the rate of the breakdown of fats rises in parallel to the rising rate of new glucose production. This rate levels off in about a week and remains high as long as we fast and maintain low insulin levels.

Some have subdivided the fasting state into three stages:

Stage 1 is the postabsorptive phase (when we quit eating) during which the brain glucose requirements are maintained by glycogen stores. We are saving some glucose by using the glycogen in the muscles instead of the glucose in the blood. This lasts about 1-2 days.

Stage 2 is from 2-10 days after eating in which new glucose is being made using amino acids secreted from the muscles, glycerol from the metabolism of triglyceride (the three fatty acids in a triglyceride molecule are connected to glycerol, and when the fatty acids are released the glycerol travels to the liver and gets converted into glucose), and pyruvate released by the muscles.

Stage 3 from day 10 onward is termed the protein conservation phase in which the fat stores are fully mobilized, and tissue use of ketones and fatty acids has increased. This is somewhat of a misnomer as growth hormone is increased by fasting and does not allow protein catabolism as much as it would if you just reduced calories. Most of the glucose comes from protein (remember now you do not need as much glucose, your brain is happy with ketones, your muscles happy with fatty acids)

As you remain fasting and lose weight, your body does catabolize the protein in your body for energy and parts. If you lost forty pounds, you would have some excess skin and you would want your body to use that extra protein. You would not need as large a heart, liver, or bones, and your body is smart enough to know that and reduce the size of these also. If you are not carrying forty extra pounds around, you may not need as large leg muscles.

I will compare this to the reduced calorie diet where these processes are different. You do not get ketogenesis, you do not markedly increase the rate of making new glucose, and you do not markedly increase the rate of using up your fat for energy and metabolizing excess protein.

You can see that in bariatric surgery, which is essentially a forced reduced calorie diet. When these people lose weight, you normally do see excess skin, and they may not have reduced their oversized internal organs as much.

In the ketogenic diet, you are taking in lots of protein as well as metabolizing your fat. Hence, you lose weight, but your body does not have any motivation to substantially reduce the excess protein in skin and organs. It can use the protein in the diet to make glucose.

Back to what is happening when you start fasting. It may appear to be counter-intuitive, but growth hormone rises after about 24 hours and continues to be elevated. You would think that it would be crazy to try to stimulate growth when no nutrients are coming in. Well, think about it. If we have no food, we need to get some. As such, we need to try to preserve the ability to obtain it. We do not want our skeletal muscles to start deteriorating as we are going to need them to run after that buffalo, or harvest some food, or walk around till we find some. Hence, despite no food coming in, we don't want to lose much muscle. Remember, if we have fat stores and stop eating, we are counting on the fat for much of the energy and are saving the muscles to eventually find food. Growth hormone also helps increase the metabolism of fat and the releasing of more fatty acids into the blood.

The same with metabolism. Your metabolism rate rises in the first days of fasting, so that you feel like you have enough energy to go find food. If not, you would spend the day napping or resting, and not out hunting.

Time to talk a little about hunger. Your body needs energy to live. Life can be boiled down to the ability to use energy, no energy, no life. As your cells and brain detect a drop in energy, mechanisms are activated to generate energy. We have already discussed the control of blood glucose and activation of fatty acids. The brain also activates the secretion of hormones that stimulate hunger. After all, eating is one of the main ways we obtain energy.

Ghrelin is a hormone secreted by the gastrointestinal tract which promotes hunger. The regulation of ghrelin fines tunes the energy requirements of the body. When ghrelin is activated, it stimulates portions of the brain that result in a desire for increased food intake. It does not necessarily increase food intake, but rather increased meals. Unlike insulin, it is secreted in a cyclical pattern which can change depending on conditions.

As we already know, hunger can be stimulated by various conditions, many of them psychological. The satisfaction of hunger also can stimulate the pleasure systems of the brain, hence the concept of comfort foods. We usually do not get hungry while sleeping and ghrelin participates in our circadian rhythms.

There is a complicated regulation of this hormone and ghrelin levels are lower in obese people as compared to leaner people. If we are fasting, we still get hungry the first couple of days around our normal mealtimes. If you are hungry and wait a couple hours, the hunger goes away. Over 2-3 days, these episodes of hunger subside so that the typical finding in those fasting is that they cease being hungry. The levels and frequency of these cyclical secretions of ghrelin subside while fasting.

Ghrelin is also associated with an increase in concentration and memory. This makes sense as when food stops coming in, we need to remember where we last saw that buffalo and figure out how to find them.

These are some of the metabolic, hormonal, and psychological effects of fasting. They begin after about six hours of no food intake but do not start reaching their full effect until about 36 hours. Once you have met your body's energy requirements by using your stored fat, it is much easier to continue with no food intake.

Now let me be clear. These metabolic changes occur with fasting. Eating once a day or snacking will place you into a reduced-calorie metabolic state, not a fasting state. The question is, why are we fasting to begin with?

I will tell you in the second half of the book about autophagy. What you need to know now is that autophagy is activated through fasting, not just only eating one meal a day. I will also go into what we are inducing when we just quit eating.

We now know more about the fasting state. I have simplified what is happening. Your body is very complex with hundreds of feedback loops requiring thousands of enzymes and is changing all the time. You are always running these programs, but the equilibrium is always changing. Even if you have been fasting for a month, you still have a little insulin floating around and there is still a little glucose being converted into fat.

There is also a difference if you are obese or nonobese. I have already advised you that if you stop eating and do not have fat stores, you are in a starvation state. If you are obese, your fasting state is somewhat different. You start with a higher baseline insulin level. If you are obese, your body has not spent a lot of time turning fat into fatty acids, in fact, it spends most of its time going in the other direction. So, it may take a little longer to get an elevation in ketones. Since your ketones do not go up as fast, it may take a little longer for your hunger to go away. No matter what, in a week you end up the same place as everyone else.

It also makes a difference if you are male or females. Females tend to go into ketosis a little faster. At the same time, female hormones tend to want to preserve fat in certain places. We know that normal females have a higher percent of body fat than males. As obesity is increased, the difference between males and females vanishes.

There really is no health reason for a non-obese person to go on an extended fast. In fact, I do not recommend this. Almost anyone can fast for a week or two without difficulty, even if you are not obese (exception something like anorexia). After that, we may get close to the starvation metabolic state which I do not recommend for anyone. Two weeks of fasting means about 10 pounds of weight. If you do not think you have 10 pounds of fat, don't fast that long.

Now I do recommend short periods of fasting. Most over four years of age should be able to fast 12 hours from the last meal at night to the next meal in the morning. All adults should be able to fast 36 hours (Eat dinner Monday, then do not eat till breakfast Wednesday) for a couple of times a week without serious consequence. These are fasts to maintain health, not to lose weight. This information does not apply to you if you have some medical condition or if you are weird.

I am now going to tell you the story of Angus who fasted for 382 days. It is interesting because he continued under medical supervision all this time and data is available.

CHAPTER 6
Angus Fast

I have included some versions of this story in most all my books as it is very instructive. First, this is an example of a fast with no caloric ingestion. He did drink coffee and bone broth and was given some extra electrolytes a couple of months, but otherwise ate noting. Taking in any calories will discount some of the effects he experienced. Also, he appeared to maintain his normal activities without difficulty. In the beginning, his goal was to reach 180 pounds. After 382 days and 276 pounds of weight loss (he started at 456 pounds), he went back to eating again. His experience is worth reading.

Angus Barbieri entered a Scottish hospital in June 1965 for a 3-week fast. He was 27 years old. At that time, he weighed 456 pounds. Fasting as a treatment for various diseases has been used for thousands of years. Angus wanted to lose weight and fasting was an appropriate treatment. After three weeks he was doing well and wanted to continue the fast. His doctors agreed and he returned to the hospital regularly over the next year. In all, he fasted for 382 days, lost 276 pounds, and stopped when he reached his goal weight of 180 pounds. One of the significant aspects of this fast is the medical documentation, and a case study was published in 1973.

Stewart, WK., Fleming, LW (1973) Features of a successful therapeutic fast of 382 days duration: Postgraduate *Medical Journal* (March 1973), *49(569), 203-209*

He lost an average of 0.7 pounds a day. During the fast, he was given vitamin supplements, and for a few months added potassium supplements. For most of the fast, his blood glucose was about 30 mg/dl. Values below 20 mg/dl were occasionally seen towards the end of the fast. There is much to take away from this fast but for our purposes a few important facts. He did not get continually hungrier throughout the fast; in fact, he reported what many others have stated that his hunger went away. His weight loss of about 0.7 pounds a day is consistent with other observations and would be considered the upper level of weight loss in fasting. He had no significant medical issues and for a short fast of a few weeks, it seems there should be no problems for most people. He was remarkably tolerant of the low glucose levels. His glucose levels were derived solely from what he was making out of protein.

Remember he started with a lot of protein as well as fat. It took a lot more tissue to support a 465-pound man versus a 180-pound man. This protein was metabolized to not only make glucose but also to provide all the minerals and electrolytes he needed. The pictures at the end do not show a man with skin sagging all over the place, but rather a normal-looking person. One can assume the excess skin was also metabolized and used as well as the excess muscle, bone, and constituents of the other organs.

A man weighing 465 pounds needs larger organs everywhere than a 180-pound man and his body was able to adjust the amount of bone, muscle heart, liver, kidney, and other organs to the appropriate size for his weight. Now, this occurred with fasting. I cannot say the same thing would occur if you were eating, such as someone who had bariatric surgery. They are not fasting but are taking in protein and carbs. There does seem to be some skin sagging on these people.

They did monitor him for a little while after he started eating. His blood sugar went back to normal.

Let me emphasize this was a fast, which is a different metabolic state than ketogenesis, which is a different metabolic state than starvation, which is a different metabolic state than a reduced calorie diet, which is a different metabolic state than a maintenance diet, which is a different metabolic state than a low carbohydrate diet.

I have found this concept to be difficult to adjust to for most people. Also fasting is a normal mechanism, not this much fasting, but certainly for a day or so. It is necessary to promote autophagy and normal homeostasis. A weight loss fast is a therapeutic fast, not a normal part of your diet. Similarly, the ketogenic diet is a weight loss diet, not a maintenance diet. Just like it would not be healthy to be on a fast all your life, it is not healthy to be in ketogenesis all your life. It is a therapeutic weight loss diet and needs to come to an end eventually.

The nerds among us can check out the case study. I picked up something when I read it again today. His cholesterol started at 230; it didn't change any. So much for the low-fat diet.

Addendum: I am still surprised at how low his blood glucose was without any symptoms. Since the normal blood glucose is around 90, it appears at least 2/3 of the energy required of the brain can be supplied by ketone bodies. It probably is more than that given that even with a low glucose level, some of that was used by other cells of the body. It could be that all the energy required by the brain can be supplied by ketones.

At the same time, I do not completely understand the glucose values. At the beginning of the fast his level was noted to be about 50 mg/dl. This is half of what a normal person should be. It did drop down to about 30 mg/dl. As I have examined other long fasts, the glucose level does drop down to about half of the original fasting level, but nobody starts at 50 mg/dl. This may be some quirk as to how they reported glucose levels fifty years ago in England. It makes more sense that his level started at 100 and dropped about half. I still can't imagine anyone walking around with a glucose of 30mg/dl. I think we can agree the level will drop 30-50%. I also think that we can agree that indeed 2/3 of the energy requirements of the grain can be provided by ketones.

I have seen (online) the post-fast pictures. You can google these also. There are no sagging body parts that you would expect with extreme weight loss. This is in marked comparison with those who have lost an equivalent percentage of fat via bariatric surgery or even with starvation. As long as you have fat stores, it appears your body can easily supply enough energy and as you lose weight, recover and reuse protein from other body parts that are getting smaller. You are metabolizing fat for energy and some of the protein for glucose. There must be some left over to maintain body structure. I know his skin surface area decreased but no sagging skin. I can only assume the skin protein was metabolized also and reused.

Also, unlike those who experience starvation, he appeared to have normal muscle mass and had no difficulty with normal activities. Those with bariatric surgery may lose an equivalent amount of weight, but they are not fasting and do get this skin sagging. Perhaps it's because these patients are taking in protein. In starvation, you are losing muscle mass, but starvation is a condition in which you have no fat stores. In studies on starvation or reduced calories, a common theme is a preoccupation with food, depression, and continuing hunger. This does not appear to be the case with fasting. There have been millions of people who have fasted for health and weight loss reasons in the last 80 years: a common theme is that hunger abates almost completely after a couple of days and energy levels remain normal.

Therapeutic fasting is a reasonable option for weight loss. Longer fasts may require some type of health care provider consultation. It's questionable if you need any extra vitamins but taking them does not seem to affect the fasting condition. I find it very unusual that health care providers never consider fasting an option for weight loss, but rather continue to repeat the vague and ineffective advice to "eat less and exercise more". We already know that the reduced calorie diet results in the worst possible consequences that would enable on to stay on a diet.

It does appear that the metabolism of excess cellular tissue, as the organ and skin structures are reduced to the appropriate size for the lower body weight, can provide the required vitamins and minerals that the body needs to remain healthy, despite the continued urinary loss. Vitamins are cheap and the doctors decided to go ahead and give him sone just to cover their liability. It is possible that the vitamins contained in the metabolized cells could have provided all he needed, but it was difficult to measure vitamin levels 45 years ago.

A brief note on the metabolic set point. As we observe in our lives, in the beginning, most people can eat whatever they want yet miraculously regulate their weight within 1-2 pounds over a year. As we get older, the weight creeps upward. I believe that means the metabolic set point creeps upward. This change in the set point probably parallels the slowing rising insulin levels from insulin resistance. It could also involve lowering growth hormones as we get older, lowering sex hormones, or some other changes in hormone levels such as thyroid. I do believe the modern western diet plays a role as this was not nearly as severe a problem (gaining weight with age) a few thousand years ago, especially if you were living for very extended periods of time. I do know that if you lose weight with most diets, if you go back to the same diet, you will gain it back.

Apparently, it is not that easy to change the set point. The Angus fast apparently did change his set point as he only gained a little more weight for the rest of his life (Five years after finishing the diet his weight was 196). It may be that fasting is the best way to change the set point. It also appears that elevated carbs may be a primary factor in raising the setpoint, and losing weight, and subsequently going on a low carb maintenance diet, may keep the set point down. There was no mention of Angus's post fast diet. I would have advised a low carb diet.

Since intermittent fasting has become popular the last few years, I again must advise you this is not a good solution to weight loss. It has been shown many times that after a short fast, you may lose weight, but usually, the weight will return. A short fast will not lower your metabolic set point. An extended fast appears to have a different effect.

Few are going to fast as long as Angus. It appears that a change in the set point will only occur in an extended fast. That is not to say fasting may not be helpful. If you are on a proper maintenance diet, adding a couple of days of fasting a month may slowly lower your metabolic set point. If you are on the normal western diet, it will not.

As above, vitamins were given during the diet. It is unknown if these were needed. Some have advised that scurvy, a lack of vitamin C, will only occur on a high carb diet. Certainly, we have evidence that the Inuit ate a diet for thousands of years with almost no fruit or vegetables. The had a low carb and high protein and fat diet. It ends up that to prevent scurvy on an almost zero carbohydrate diet, you only need about 10 mg of Vitamin Ca day. Most animals make their own Vitamin C and just eating animals can provide you with plenty.

Now you must eat the meat raw or barely cooked as heat destroys Vitamin C. Examination of these diets also show that the maximum amount of protein that was comfortably eaten was about one third, an observation that has been noted in other cultures (including ours), and that about 35-40% protein is the max tolerated. You can see these people ate about 50-60% fat. A very high protein diet can be dangerous, and there was evidence that hunters discarded animals with little fat; even when food was scarce. A protein only diet leads to nausea, diarrhea, wasting, and death.

Since there was little vegetable or fruit, you can see the other vitamins were also provided by the meat. It is quite likely that Angus did not need the extra vitamins as he could have scavenged them from the self-protein he was metabolizing. I can see the point of covering your ass by giving him vitamins. They were cheap and did not have any calories, so why take the risk.

As an aside, it appears that you increase your need for Vitamin C if you eat carbohydrates. We are acquainted with scurvy from sailors at sea for months. We know that carbohydrates are the easiest food to store for times of scarcity, and these sailors ate mainly carbs and protein on these long trips. Not only that, but they also cooked most of the Vitamin C containing foods, which inactivated the vitamin.

Of course, most people, Inuit or not, are now on some form of the western diet and now get the associated western diet diseases. If you provide it to them, people want to eat junk food.

Angus was also given potassium supplements Day 3 to Day 162 based on a low serum level (the only one) on day 93. Again, he had no symptoms, and we still don't know if he needed it, but we had to cover our ass.

Therapeutic fast is a weight loss diet. After a reasonable weight loss has been obtained, you go on a maintenance diet. If you go back to your previous diet, you will regain the weight. I do not know what diet Angus went on after he lost weight. I believe it is very likely he changed his set point and went on a normal diet instead of his previous high carb diet. His parents owned a fish&chips booth where he worked, and I am guessing his previous diet was all the fish and chips he could eat. After he lost weight, he moved to a different city.

Fasting can be added to the low carb diet. The low carb diet is what you must be on to control your glucose levels and it is a maintenance diet, not a weight loss diet. It is quite likely you will lose some weight. If you desire to lose more weight (keep it to a reasonable amount, not your 18 y/o weight), you can always add a few days of fasting now and then.

In general, exercise is not a good weight loss strategy. It does increase hunger. It does increase calorie expenditure. But the number of increased calories expended is minor compared to the number of calories expended just to keep you alive. You can swim for an hour, but if you eat an extra piece of toast, you almost gain those calories back. I don't know about you, but I get hungry after an hour of swimming.

To use exercise as a weight loss strategy, you must do a lot. I'm talking about 5-7 miles walking/running a day. You can lose weight through exercise, but if you have a job it takes up all your extra time. As you get older, injuries start to occur, and you have difficulty maintaining that level of exercise. Diet is the overriding factor in weight loss for most people. If you use exercise as your weight loss program, like all other weight-loss diets, you eventually must go on a maintenance diet.

There is a minor place for exercise in prediabetes and diabetes. Exercise will increase the amount of glucose absorbed by muscle, even in the absence of insulin. You may be lowering your insulin requirement (and saving money if you are on insulin) if you exercise. But again, this pales in comparison to decreased carbohydrate ingestion.

Next chapter a slightly different fast. I will add this because it is a more modern case review and thus had more blood tests done. It will also demonstrate that not all extended fasts are the same.

The next chapter is for nerds. If you don't like biochemistry, skip the chapter. I will not go into detailed explanations of biochemistry as I don't have enough time. I imagine this will only be of interest to less than 5% of the readers of this book. I include this chapter because I am a nerd, and since I am also the editor of the book, I get to do what I want.

CHAPTER 7
Nerd Fast

I will go through a forty-day fast which had been recorded as a clinical study. I realize this hardly compares with Angus's fast, but it does get us into Stage 3 of fasting. This study was done about 10 years after that fast and a few more laboratory tests were done.

The first thing to recognize is that this patient was not obese with a BMI of 23. As time has gone on, we recognize that the metabolism of the obese is not the same as a nonobese person. You simply can't apply the same parameters. The data we gathered on Angus may be like any obese person on a prolonged therapeutic fast but will vary from that of the nonobese.

We should never see a prolonged therapeutic fast in the nonobese and I do not advise that at all. Nevertheless, it is interesting to see some of the differences. This patient was a 41 y/o monk who was undergoing a religious fast and consented to be medically monitored. He planned for a 40 day fast. He had previously been on a diet of vegetables, eggs, and milk products. Physically he was in normal condition except for sinus bradycardia with a rate of 45-50

To start with, he only lasted 36 days until profound weakness and symptoms of postural hypotension interfered with his daily activities. Already this is different from Angus who lasted ten times as long and had no problems with his daily activities during the 382 days of his fast. At the start, this patient appeared to be in normal if not good physical condition. A BMI of 23 puts you in the normal category, which means you probably had at least 15 pounds of stored fat. Using Angus (obese) weight loss average, that would give you about 21 days' worth of fat storage.

This is an interesting observation in itself. I have told you that no one should have problems with a couple of weeks of fasting. I may have to revise that statement by saying no one with a normal BMI should have a problem. Maybe if you are normal, you should limit a prolonged fast to three weeks. If you are thin, maybe one week.

Over the 36 days fast he lost about 0.9 pounds a day compared with Angus 0.7 pounds. We now realize that an obese person exerts a lot of energy just carrying that extra 250 pounds around. We also know that the obese may have a slightly lower relative metabolic set point. I told you before that it is difficult to change this set point.

Usually, we eat around a million calories a year (active adult male). Most young people can maintain their weight without any difficulty; that is, they eat whatever they want, and their weight is constant. If you need more energy, your body makes you hungry. If you need less, you are not hungry. That is, simply eating when you are hungry and not eating when you are not, enables you to almost balance this calorie load exactly.

If we assume a pound of fat has 3500 calories, that means if you ate just 0.35% more calories a year you would gain one pound a year. Your metabolic set point controls your calorie intake and keeps you from getting fat unless something goes wrong. I will address what goes wrong in the last chapter.

Anyway, I am going to assume this patient had a somewhat higher relative metabolic set point and hence may have lost weight at a little faster rate than Angus. As I said, nonobese should not have prolonged fasts so I am still going to say that 0.7 pounds a day is the average weight loss.

This patient had to stop the diet early secondary to postural hypotension. Although Angus did not have his blood pressure or pulse recorded, we know through other studies that prolonged diets typically result in a fall in both blood pressure and pulse, setting someone up for postural hypotension. I will discuss the diuresis that occurs with weight loss in a minute but let us remind ourselves that Angus did not have this problem.

There was also a slight difference in their fasts. Although we said this patient was fasting, he was taking in 60 calories from daily communion a day (15 grams carb). This then was not a fast, and may have reduced some of the accommodations of the body in a total fast. He really was on a reduced calorie diet (very reduced calorie) and hence had some elements of this type of diet which may have reduced his capacity to fast no more than 36 days.

It has been consistently shown that salt and water loss in fasting, and to some extent in the ketogenic diet, increases, and peaks 3-4 days after starting the diet. This explains the common finding in almost any diet that you lose weight at the start. Of course, this is water weight (8.3 pounds per gallon), and your body is about 55% water.

This increased water loss has been explained by changes in hormones, but we believe it is mainly due to increases in ketones. For your kidney to get rid of ketones (which are negatively charged), it must have a positively charged ion with it. Initially, this is a sodium ion. So as the ketones increase, the amount of sodium excreted also increases, reaching a peak sodium excretion after about three days and then diminishing to normal at the two-week mark. To excrete this sodium, water must also be lost, hence the initial increased weight loss.

If we recall, during the first part of fasting, after the glycogen has been used up, the liver and kidney have been using protein and amino acids to make glucose. The result of the metabolism of protein is the generation of an ammonia cation (NH_2) which is positive, and this replaces the sodium ion. After two weeks the sodium excretion is back to normal, and the ammonia excretion is elevated.

Rising glucagon and falling insulin also contribute to the early phase of diuresis as this combination increases sodium excretion.

In this patient, the sodium level gradually fell somewhat. With Angus, it remained constant. One reason for this may be that Angus drank noncaloric bone broth with is a good source of electrolytes. He also was completely fasting which may have prevented some of the hypotensive effects this patient had on his very reduced calorie diet. In any case, it probably is wise to drink bone broth or some other noncaloric electrolytic solution. Remember, this guy did not even make it to his 40-day goal secondary to postural hypotension, whereas Angus went as long as he wanted.

At this point, I will examine in a little more detail Stage 2 of fasting. Skip this section unless you are a nerd. As you will recall, when we stop eating, the liver maintains blood glucose (mainly for the brain) by releasing glucose from the glycogen stores. At the same time, the liver begins increasing its manufacturing of new glucose in the liver. The liver is always making new glucose and is in equilibrium with the requirements. If the insulin level is high (and glucagon is low), it does not have to make a lot of glucose. If the opposite situation is present, it ramps up production.

Although the glycogen in the liver only lasts about a day, your blood sugar rarely drops so low if affects your thinking. Most of the time you will be eating again in 12 hours anyway. If you go longer than 12 hours without eating, we are counting on that new glucose production more.

If you recall, the muscles of your body also contain glycogen with can be converted into glucose. This glucose cannot be secreted into the blood, so it does not help your brain much. It does conserve a little of the blood glucose by using the muscle's own glycogen.

All this time we are waiting for the metabolism of our stored fat to ramp up. We know that once we release enough fatty acids and the liver converts these into ketones, we will have plenty of energy and the brain will be able to get most of its energy from the ketones and not have to rely on blood glucose as much. It appears that even in fasting, your blood glucose does not go to zero. There are a few tissues in the body that also must use glucose for energy. The brain seems to be able to function fine using at least 70% ketones for energy.

It takes longer to get fatty acids released and converted into ketones than just to release glycogen from the liver, and we need that new glucose from the liver quickly.

Enter the Cori cycle. The muscle can use this stored glycogen and break it down to provide energy to make the muscle work. If there is plenty of oxygen around, it usually breaks it down completely via the citric acid cycle. If there is not enough oxygen or the insulin level is down and glucagon is up, the muscle only breaks the glucose down into pyruvate.

Pyruvate is the earliest product of glucose metabolism and contains three carbon atoms. This can then be entered into the citric acid cycle to make lots of energy, or converted back into glucose, or converted to a fatty acid, or used to make alanine, another type of amino acid.

Of course, all these other uses (other than the citric acid cycle) require energy, and the reason we broke down the glucose in the first place was to get energy for the muscle. The pyruvate can be rapidly converted to lactate. Many of us are familiar with lactic acid buildup in muscle during strenuous activity. In general, we do not like this to happen and would rather enough oxygen be supplied to the muscle to prevent this.

At the start of fasting, the muscle releases this lactate (which originated in the muscle glycogen) into the blood where it is taken up by the liver. The liver than reverses this process and converts 2 lactates into 2 pyruvates into glucose. This new glucose can then be put into the blood for anyone (brain) to use.

You don't get something for nothing. You get two ATP molecules (stored energy) for the muscles when you break down the glycogen into glucose into pyruvate, but it costs the liver 6 ATP molecules to convert the lactate back to glucose. So, you lose energy every time you do this.

Your body has determined that it is worth it to make new glucose to keep your brain happy. It turns out that this is quite important to bridge the Stage 2 to Stage 3 fasting gap. After 12 hours of fasting, new glucose made by the liver accounts for about 40% of the glucose. After 24 hours about 70%, and after 40 hours about 90%. You can see the glycogen runs out not too long after starting fasting. After 12 hours, the Cori cycle accounts for about 20% of the new glucose, after 24 hours this about doubles.

The Cori cycle involves the muscle metabolism of glycogen into pyruvate, the pyruvate going to lactate, the lactate secreted into the blood where it is taken up by the liver (and kidney), this is then converted back into pyruvate and then onto glucose which is secreted back into the blood.

You can see the Cori cycle is important in the 12-48 hour fasting time to help ensure there is enough glucose around till the ketones ramp up production. This process also conserves protein catabolism in the body. We are trying to conserve out muscles and do not want them used just to make glucose if possible. The Cori cycle not only provides a rapid substrate for making new glucose, but it also keeps us from using up our protein. As the fat cells break down triglycerides to fatty acids, the left-over glycerol is also used by the liver to make glucose.

Even though we have the Cori cycle and the lactate coming from the muscle, about 10% of the new glucose from early fasting comes from protein-derived amino acids. It ends up that alanine is the main amino acid released by muscles. It appears that the muscles increase production of this amino acid and release it into the blood to be used by the liver to make more glucose. Please note, I have saying that the liver is making new glucose, but the kidneys to a lesser extent are also doing the same thing.

When you are making glucose out of amino acids, you will have a nitrogen group left over which is converted into urea and excreted out the kidney. It also appears that the branched-chain amino acids are preferably metabolized in the muscle to provide nitrogen to make alanine from pyruvate. This may seem to be unnecessarily complicated, but like a lot of processes in the human body, this provides mechanisms for feedback inhibition. Rising insulin inhibits new glucose by preventing alanine uptake by the liver.

Ketones inhibit new glucose by decreasing catabolism of branched amino acids, thus eliminating the nitrogen source to make alanine. About 99.99% of the time when you start this process you are going to start eating soon. Most of the time you will not be going on to fasting, and we do not want too much glucose, which may happen if you are making a lot and eating a lot.

There are many of you out there on metformin for your type 2 diabetes. The way this drug keeps your glucose down is by inhibiting the liver from making new glucose. So, you can see that given the go-ahead, your liver can make lots of glucose. If you inhibit the liver from making glucose out of lactate, the lactate can build up. Usually, you can just get rid of it through the kidney, but if your kidneys are not working well, you can get lactic acidosis. That is why we usually check your kidney function before putting you on metformin.

You remember that if we quit eating (start fasting), that we want to save our muscles so we can go out and get more food. We had to sacrifice a little protein for the first couple of days to tide our glucose over and make our brain happy. As the ketones rise, protein catabolism is inhibited, which is OK because our brain is now using ketones and we don't need as much new glucose. This happens more rapidly for an obese person than one with a normal BMI, as we may be able to go one for a long time with all that stored energy, and we want to save muscle. Again, we are looking at fasting in obese vs. nonobese, there is a difference.

The rate of metabolism of fat with the release of fatty acids, as well as the rate of the formation of new ketones by the liver, rises to a maximum in about three days and then remains steady. If we happened to be measuring ketones in the blood, we would see the ketone level rise for three to four weeks. What's with that.

It turns out that the uptake of ketones by the muscles decreases quite a bit, as energy for muscle metabolism shifts from ketones to free fatty acids. This is quite handy as your brain cannot use fatty acids for energy (the molecules are too large to get into the brain), so as our fasting continues and our glucose level drops, it leaves plenty of ketones for the brain, and our muscles are happy to use the fatty acids. Your brain is very selfish and will gladly take energy from your other organs. It is also handy that as your ketones increase, it inhibits catabolism of protein to make more glucose. We want to save muscles and by now your brain does not need nearly as much glucose. We have plenty of fatty acids to go around for everyone else.

Let me mention growth hormone again. I told you that it rises with fasting. It does, but growth hormone is also affected by lots of different things, and it also is secreted in a pulsatile manner. It does go up in fasting and I told you that this was to help preserve muscles, but perhaps it is equally important in making sure your glucose levels do not go too low. Under certain conditions, growth hormone can increase blood sugar, and this is an example of your body's often complicated and redundant regulatory mechanisms.

I'll talk about fasting and thyroid in a later chapter.

Mineral balance in fasting is quite variable and changes as the fast goes on. We already talked about how sodium is being lost early on, but the plasma sodium levels are constant. Potassium also changes throughout. In this patient, it remained stable. In Angus, it fell for a few months and then went back to normal. The source of potassium may be from the catabolism of other body parts as your body adjusts the size of your body from the weight loss. Of course, Angus had some potassium replacement pills for a couple of months, but the doctors were just treating the lab test and he had no symptoms.

For short fasting (two weeks) I do not think we need to pay any attention to electrolytes or minerals if you are a normal person. For prolonged therapeutic fasting, we could just do what Angus did and take bone broth or supplements; as long as there are no calories, take what you want. This is a therapeutic fast to lose fat and we also want you to be in good health. We are not trying to prove anything.

Calcium is also all over the map. You, of course, have all the calcium you want in your bones. As Angus lost the 276 pounds, he did not need as much bone and his body gradually remodeled them and used the calcium as needed. Magnesium, Zinc, and Phosphorus have also been measured in various fasts and no particular problems have arisen. Some of these minerals are being recovered from bone and the catabolism of other body parts such that replacement does not seem to be required.

Uric acid is somewhat more complicated. It does seem to rise in fasting, then levels out but at a somewhat higher level. Why this occurs is not certain. It may relate to decreased uric acid excretion during fasting as uric acid and keto acids may compete for the same renal tubular transport sites. In any case, this may increase the risk of uric acid stones. I advise people to drink a lot of water while fasting for several reasons. It does seem to lessen hunger if that should arise, especially early on. As I just said, it may reduce the risk of uric acid stones by diluting the urine more.

Also, although this is hard to prove, it may dilute whatever toxins are being released by the fat. Modern man gets a lot of environmental toxins. Your body tries to protect you by storing some of the fat-soluble ones in your fat tissue. As you lose fat, these toxins are released. We want to dilute them and get them out of us through the urine if possible. Drink a lot of water or any noncaloric fluid. You can drink diet drinks if necessary. Usually, I eventually advise people to cut back on artificially sweetened drinks. It has been shown that they do not particularly help with weight loss. They do desensitize the taste buds to sweet and makes you desire more. They are also likely to adversely affect your gut biome.

A therapeutic fast is a somewhat desperate measure. You have already failed at lesser treatments. It is worth the risk of diet drinks to get you to stay on the fast and potentially change your metabolic set point. That will give us a chance to get you on the right maintenance diet and we can talk about those diet drinks in a later chapter.

Prolonged fasts are different in obese and nonobese.

Prolonged fasts are different in men and women.

A reduced calorie diet (even very reduced) is not the same as fasting.

Many of these changes in metabolism occur in the ketogenic diet but this diet is not the same as fasting. Eating anything, even just protein (which I do not advise) takes you out of fasting and affects some of your body's adaptation to that condition.

Kerndt PR, Naughton JL, Driscoll CE, et al.
Fasting: The History, Pathophysiology and Complications,
Western Journal of Medicine
1982 NOV;137.379-399

CHAPTER 8
Risks of Fasting

DO NOT DO ANY EXTENED FASTING TILL YOU READ THIS CHAPTER.

Fasting for 2-3 weeks should be benign for a normal person. If you are at all not normal, and some people are not normal, you should see a real doctor, or at least talk to them. If you are taking medications, then that complicates the situation, and you may have to see someone.

I'm not talking about the normal 12 hours fast or those who fast a couple of nonconsecutive days a week, but for those who want to go on a therapeutic diet. These people are all obese, or should be, to go on this diet. I do not advise the starvation metabolic state, so don't start if you don't have fat. Also, your goal needs to be reasonable, not your weight when you were eighteen.

You must do the 12 hours fast. I highly encourage occasionally not eating for a day (that is skipping breakfast, lunch, and dinner). Almost no harm should come to a normal person by doing that.

There have been reports of fatalities using therapeutic fasting. In the Angus case study, they reported that they could find five fatalities in the medical literature. One was attributed to lactic acidosis during the refeeding period. Two were ventricular failure at 3 weeks and 8 weeks into the fast. Both of these had shown evidence of heart failure before starting the fast. One patient died on the thirteenth day of the fast from small bowel obstruction.

The fifth was associated with a fast of more than 200 days. It occurred during refeeding of a young woman and may have been associated with allopurinol which had been given.

Let us remember these patients had morbid obesity at the start.

Others have reported a death on day 13 of renal failure. Subsequent chronic glomerulonephritis was found at autopsy.

Another case involved a patient who was otherwise in good health and had been given small amounts of protein supplements (essential amino acids) for 103 days of a 210 day fast. He died of intractable ventricular arrhythmias on the eighth day of refeeding. This case demonstrates what we already knew. Protein supplements during fasting have been implicated in several fasting deaths. Often with the refeeding and almost always with heart problems.

I do not advise protein supplements (especially liquid) to be used with any fasting protocol. First, it is not a fast if you take in calories. It appears a very reduced calorie diet may be far more dangerous than a fast. Consider the monk in the previous chapter. Instead of a fast, he was on a reduced calorie diet. Second, liquid protein diets have been associated with numerous deaths, mainly from ventricular arrhythmias, and I advise avoiding this completely. This does not appear to be a problem with the ketogenic diet, but still avoid protein supplements.

Other problems include gout, postural hypotension, and arrhythmias.

We must pay attention to the re-eating phase of the fast. You can see that two of the five deaths in the Angus paper occurred during the refeeding phase as did the death in the previous paragraph.

Carbohydrate refeeding after fasting produces a sharp weight gain with immediate reversal of urinary salt and water loss and can result in obvious edema. Refeeding with fat does not do this. When refeeding, we should start with small amounts of fat and protein. When you stop the diet, you are not very hungry. Do not go to the all- you- can- eat buffet.

Bottom line do not eat during a fast. Then it is not a fast. Avoid all liquid protein. Drink a lot. Be careful when you start eating again.

CHAPTER 9
Different Fasts

Just like diets and metabolic states, it seems to be our nature to subdivide subjects and give them names. So it is with fasts. Let's be clear, fasting is not taking in any calories and does not require much instruction. Just don't eat. Some people believe that fasting also involves no fluid intake. Do not do that. The only time this should occur if for religious fasts, or maybe just before surgery. Anytime I say fast it means no calories, but lots of fluids.

I will mention again the 12 hours fast. It appears we may have been created to eat after the sun comes up and before the sun goes down. In the last couple hundred years in response to extending the workday with lighting, we now eat three times a day.

Regardless, it is important for healthy homeostasis to fast 12 hours between the last meal of the day and the first of the next day. The absence of this simple habit may be contributing to our current obesity epidemic.

Since this is not a fast but a normal pattern, I am not going to call it a fast. It is just a normal life.

We divide up fasts into three categories:

Intermittent Fasting. These are fasts lasting up to two days that can be done weekly. We often use this to maintain weight or perhaps as a part of a diet to lose weight. These can be from not eating after dinner, skip eating the next day, and then eat breakfast the following day. This ends up being a 36 hour fast. This time frame is important as we will see when we talk about autophagy. It appears that if you skip eating one day, you may eat slightly more when you start eating again, but not twice as much. This fast is not done on consecutive days.

Periodic fasting: These are fasts lasting at least two days but no longer than 2 weeks. As with intermittent fasting, medical risks are very low. Usually, this is done with a specific goal in mind. You may be fasting to help a medical problem. You may fast to achieve a work or personal goal. Maybe you fast just to demonstrate to yourself the power of self-will. Maybe you are going on a business trip for a few days, and you want to save money by not buying any food. Some people on diets may have trouble obtaining the right food in restaurants and it is much easier just not to eat. It is much easier and better for you if you just skip eating rather than go on some type of short-term reduced calorie diet.

Therapeutic Fasting: These fasts last 3 weeks or longer and are almost always done for weight loss. Often these are people who have failed everything else, and this is a last resort. Of course, you may just have a bride who is trying to lose 10 quick pounds to get into a wedding dress. She should be able to fast 2-3 weeks, lose that weight, and have no problems with the wedding. This is really a much better option than going on a reduced calorie diet and exercising a lot more. You will only be hungry for a couple of days. You will free up time to prepare for the wedding. And you will have a much better mental state. These people are often motivated and have no problems.

These are the general classes of fasting. With our previous knowledge, we recognize the Stage 1 metabolic state is present with intermittent fasting, Intermittent fasting is also involved in the Stage 2 metabolic state, and Stage 3 is the therapeutic fasting state. With these three categories, we go through three different metabolic states, all distinct. Now let us examine the common fasts, mainly intermittent, that have their own names.

16:8 Fast: Every 24 hours you spend 8 hours eating and 16 hours fasting. Although this does not appear to be a real fast, it may be a good idea. In my other books, I have emphasized that insulin resistance may be the basis for our diabetic and obesity epidemics. I believe it is the multiple episodes of insulin elevations that are the main factor.

The modern diet is characterized by frequent between-meal eating. Just eating a few times a day may help a lot. This fast may just involve skipping breakfast every day and keeping the 12 hours fast at night.

20:4 fast: This is also called the Warrior Diet and it makes sense. Probably many have eaten this way for a while. It may occur in wartime, but it also may occur in several jobs. The advantage is that you would have a hard time eating too much. You also would not have to worry about between-meal snacks. Some use this fast on Thanksgiving Day. Don't eat dinner the day before, don't start eating till noon, then eat all you want for the next four hours. Do not eat again till breakfast the next day.

OMAD fast: This is one meal a day. Usually, this meal is dinner. Eat dinner today, then do not eat till dinner tomorrow. Again, this lets you avoid between-meal snacks and multiple elevations of insulin. You, of course, do not eat after dinner and you maintain you 12 hours fast. You can always do this on your maintenance diet by just skipping breakfast and lunch. As time goes on, you are not afraid of not eating. If you skipped breakfast and got a little hungry at lunch but were too busy, just fast till dinner. By now you know that hunger only lasts about an hour and then goes away. By now you are not worried about a little hunger. You appreciate your ghrelin elevation.

5:2 fast: This is also called the Fast Diet and has become quite popular. You eat your normal diet 5 days a week and don't eat two days a week. Please use this with your normal 12 hours fast. Also, do not do this on consecutive days. You can do this with whatever diet you are on now, be it low carb, low fat, high fat, or even reduced calorie. It is also quite flexible as you pick the days. People usually use this for weight loss or weight maintenance. I encourage you to begin this after dinner, skip all the next day's meals, eat breakfast the day after. Now it is a 36 hour fast. This diet will be more effective for weight loss if you are on the maintenance diet.

I have written much about the maintenance diet, a diet for the entire family which you do for fifty years. This fast allows different individuals to just skip eating themselves and let everyone else eat normally. If you are trying to lose a little weight, you can do this on your own without putting extra work on the food engineer.

There is a variation of this diet whereby people just eat fewer calories on the fast days. Don't do this. You are now on the worst diet, that being the reduced calorie diet and you forgo all the benefits of fasting. Everyone(99.99% of us) should be able to not eat a day. I will talk about the fear of starvation later. It is a mental state that can be overcome.

Thyroid Fast: This fast alternates fasting with feasting. Take two days a week where you do not eat and eat all you want the day after. This fast is designed to help the thyroid cycle its output. Insulin facilitates the conversion of T4 to T3. In fasting, T4 goes down and T3 remains the same. Eventually, TSH goes down. In my book on the ketogenic diet in which insulin is down, I do advise people to get out of ketosis every 3 weeks for a day or two by eating a high carbohydrate meal. Insulin is involved in other hormone production and continuous low insulin levels may affect sex hormones. On the ketogenic diet, it only takes a day or two to get back into ketosis.

Water fast: This just means you drink water (or some other non-caloric liquid) during your fast. All fasts should be water fasts. You should not only be drinking liquids; you should be drinking more liquids than usual. A religious fast may not allow any liquids, but this is a special case.

Keto Reset Diet: This is just a low carb diet with a few food recommendations. Essentially a ketogenic diet.

Metabolism Reset Diet: This is also just a ketogenic diet.

Therapeutic Fasts are rare.

Periodic Fast are also rare.

Intermittent Fasts are the ones you are going to either do or run across. I have already advised you that I think fasting is part of the normal homeostasis of humans since the beginning. These are intermittent Fasts. Do not count that 12 hour fast as a fast. It is just normal life.

It may be difficult for you to believe but eventually, I will convince you to fast a little. Maybe only 24 hours, but I am almost sure you will do it. Maybe just to prove to yourself you can.

CHAPTER 10
Fear of Fasting

For no man ever hated his oven flesh; but nourished and cherisheth it,

> *even as the Lord the Church:*
> *Ephesians 5:6*

Man seems to have an innate fear of fasting. Upon reflection, maybe it's a fear of starvation. I have experienced seeing this fear when I have discussed fasting with people. Almost everyone agrees that going a couple of days without eating is not going to harm you, yet everyone says I am crazy if I ask them to fast. It seems more instinctual that logical.

I imagine this was not the case throughout human history, as having to skip a meal or two may have been a common event. Man probably did not like it, but they were not afraid of it. There was still probably a fear of starvation, but most understood if they ran out of food, they would have a few days to get some more without harming themselves.

In the modern world, we can now get food delivered to our door 24 hours a day, seven days a week. The grocery store is open 24 hours, and the local convenience store is only 5 minutes away. The fear of not eating for a few days has vanished. Perhaps modern man is so conditioned to having food readily available that the thought of not eating is frightening. Even in ancient Egyptian times, if you had money, you could get food, even if there was a famine. I wonder if they were also afraid of fasting.? Does the thought of fasting unconsciously stir some primal fear of starvation?

Throughout history, fasting was used as a treatment for disease. This may have been a chronic disease, or maybe you just had an upset stomach. Advising one to fast was not crazy, but more likely common medical advice. Has your health care provider ever advised you to fast?

If you and your friends were stuck in a cabin because of a blizzard and had no food, would the first reaction be "Oh no. What are we going to do?" Or would it be "no big deal. We just won't eat for a few days". I think you know what the answer would be.

Before I go on, I will admit that you will be hungry when you fast. You will also get sore if you exercise or have a little pain in you get operated on. We expect that and can live with it. We do not like fear of the unknown. I often have told someone that if I do this it may hurt a little. They still let me do it. By the way, if someone tells you it may hurt a little, that means it may hurt a lot.

Your cyclic secretion of ghrelin will remind you that it is dinnertime and if you are fasting, you will get a little hungry. If you wait a little, the hunger will go away. The more times this happens, the less you fear it. As time goes on the ghrelin secretion decreases and you do not even remember it's mealtime. This seems to be a common experience, that is you get progressively less hungry when fasting till after a couple days you do not notice it. Otherwise, how could someone fast for 382 days.

Now if you are on a reduced calorie diet or starving (no fat stores), that is not the case. Your hunger continues after a couple days and gets worse. You spend your time thinking about food and it occupies your dreams. It does not go away. I have tried to emphasize this point throughout; fasting is a unique metabolic state and is different from just reducing the number of calories you eat.

When fasting, after the hunger fades, your energy seems to go up. Upon measuring the basal metabolic rate, it goes up after 24 hours, and at 72 hours it is at least 10% above normal. Later, you will see this does not appear to be a direct result of the thyroid levels and appears to be more related to other changes in the hormonal milieu.

You are still somewhat hungry after 1-2 days, but that is understandable as it may take that long for us to get full transition to the increased levels of fatty acids and ketones as the glucose level starts to drop. You remember our talk about inducing various cellular processes. The more often you fast, the more rapidly this adjustment occurs, and the less time you have feeling tired or hungry.

But let's be real. A little hunger is to be expected when you start to fast. Your body is supposed to notify you when your energy supplies are dropping. In our conscious mind we know that we really have plenty of energy in our fat, it is just going to take a little while before we get access to it via the generation of fatty acids and ketones. You may try drinking liquids to fool your stomach, or caffeine to up your adrenaline a little (no hunger when the bear is chasing you), but as time has gone on, I've decided to just tell people to "Suck it up". Lately I've changed that to "Gird up you loins" ,as too many people though I was referring to cocaine which does decrease your hunger.

In any case, there are many situations in life where you must do things you may be afraid to do. From asking someone on a date to a job interview to running a 5K: the first time you do it is the hardest and it gets easier the more times you do it. At least with fasting this is not all psychological. The more often you fast, the more you induce your metabolism to switch over to ketosis more rapidly. Also, it's hard to have your first child. By the third at least you know the pain will stop.

Before I go on, I must discuss the maintenance diet a little. The rising incidence of Obesity, Diabetes, and Prediabetes can be mainly attributed to the modern western diet. There may be a few other more minor influences, but I can get most people to agree to that premise.

The solution is to change the diet. This is not as simple as it sounds. For the last 75 years, the government has been in the business of giving you advice on your diet. This has been a colossal failure. The advancement of processed food and advertising has further contributed to the failing health of western countries. Don't tell me we have much better health now. We may have much better science, but the life span has not changed that much, whereas the portion of our life we live with disabilities has increased. We no longer are healthy till we die, but rather a third of our life is spent in poor health.

I have written two books on the maintenance diet. As you may guess, fasting is a part of this diet. Do not worry, I am not talking about fasting for a few months; but not eating for 36 or up to 72 hours a couple of times a year should not scare you, although right now it probably does.

Up to this point, I have given you some idea as to what happens when you fast. Sure, I used Angus's fast as a dramatic example and looked at the monk's very reduced calorie diet (not exactly a fast), but no one reading this book is going to go to that extent. It does serve as an example of what happens in a fast, even for a couple of days, and I give these examples to diminish your fear of fasting.

I have also emphasized not eating for 12 hours between dinner and breakfast. If I don't call it a fast, more people would be comfortable doing this. Just to be clear, this means you do not take in any calories for 12 hours. If you have a midnight snack one night or go to the movies and get a bag of popcorn, you may have to skip breakfast the next morning to get in the 12 hours.

I'm sure at one time in your life you have skipped breakfast. Maybe you accidentally fasted 16 hours. With just a little self-confidence you could skip lunch and not eat till dinner. Remember you hunger will go away in about an hour and think of how the ghrelin is helping you think. Before you know it, you have fasted 24 hours. And this was mainly by accident. All I have to do is get you to skip dinner and voila, we have 36 hours of fasting, and on our way to the 5:2 fast.

I do not expect this to happen right away. I do expect you to institute the 12 hours fast tonight It will not take that long for this to be a normal part of your life. You will skip breakfast someday and remember this paragraph. If you are feeling good about yourself, you may just ride it out till the next day.

Everyone who fasts says it gets easier after you have done it a few times. Generally, they are speaking about the several days fast, but even the 36 hours fast gets easier. I think the 36 hours fast getting easier is mostly psychological, as you have just started that metabolic adjustment and your fatty acids have not gone up enough. The few days fast may be a greater physiologic effect, as by now you have lots of energy for your body to use. Your metabolism is up, your energy supply is up, your human growth hormone is up, and your leptin is down.

Almost all of you will try the 12 hours fast between the last and first meal. It is probably part of our basic homeostasis throughout history for us to do that. There will be some who will do the one meal a day. It really involves only skipping breakfast and lunch, and many of you have done that already. There will be some who will go the 36 hours. Many of these will have read about the maintenance diet and are interested in a lifetime of good health.

There will be some who try to fast for a week or so. They are probably ae not doing this to lose weight, but more of a confidence builder to see if they can. These are the same people who run a marathon. Not to win, but to prove to themselves that they can do it.

Eventually you are no longer bound by your eating habits. You may find skipping eating a day to just be too convenient. Going on a plane trip, it can be much less stressful not to worry about eating on the plane, in the airport, at the hotel that evening, if you just skip eating that day. For you it would be no big deal. N:ow you are not going to panic if you are snowed in a cabin deep in the woods and there is no food. If you have water, you are not going to do anything crazy.

This is a book about fasting, but subtlety I am herding you toward a lifetime maintenance diet that includes fasting.

I added a chapter at the end of this book in which I fasted for 28 days (really 27 days) I go into more detail as to what causes hunger. You may want to skip to the back and read this chapter.

CHAPTER 11
The Gut Microbiome

This seems to be a reasonable spot to talk about the gut microbiome. It seems strange but fasting affects this. Lots of things affect your microbiome, and as time goes on, we are beginning to realize that disease and your gut microbiome are very interconnected.

First, what is your gut microbiome? These are all the organisms living peacefully inside of you. Not inside of you, but just like your skin separates the outside world from your inside, the gut also separates outside from inside. Its job is much more complicated as it must let some stuff into your body while keeping other stuff out. About half of your stool is composed of microorganisms. Almost all your energy is absorbed through your gut. Your gut breaks down food as I have described earlier, but after breaking it down, it must sift through the contents and absorb what we want. It must also keep what we don't want out.

The gut microbiome is the accumulation of bacteria, fungi, viruses, and parasites that live in our digestive tract. This composition varies all the time, and portions can persist for many years (some a lifetime) It is different in different parts of the world, different parts of the United States, different parts of your city, and even different parts of your neighborhood. We are certain it plays a vital role in the immune system response to various antigens. We believe it plays a role in obesity and diabetes. It almost certainly plays a role in autoimmune diseases such as rheumatoid arthritis. The gut biome aids in the digestion of food, synthesizes various products import to us (vitamins), prevents the growth of pathogenic organisms, and maybe communicates with our brain.

You get your first dose at your birth, and it makes a difference whether it is vaginal or via c-section. Of course, your parents contribute to this in early life (breast or bottle feeding is different). Your pets contribute their share as do the various products you put in your mouth while a toddler (toys, dirt, bugs, whatever is on the floor). You can see your diet contributes quite a bit. We say your stomach sterilizes the food you eat, but we say that to make us feel better. Various organisms are protected from the acid by coverings. Fiber can form a gel in the stomach protecting other organisms. Sometimes things pass rapidly through the stomach and not enough time is available to sterilize anything. I still say the stomach sterilizes food when it suits me, like when I pick something off the floor and eat it.

I'm pretty sure that as we get better at identifying all the organisms, no two people will be exactly the same. I made digestion sound simple, but your body is not 100% efficient at absorbing all the nutrients you get. Some get through the body and feeds this massive population of organisms. (More organisms than cells in your body.)

The change in the microbiome is just another example of how your body can adjust to your environment to keep you alive and well. If you move, the biome changes a little because the food may have changed a little. If you have a poor diet, the biome changes in your body's attempt to keep you well, but that may not keep you healthy.

Most of us are somewhat familiar with skin bacteria (part of the skin microbiome) We know that some bacteria are normal, and their growth inhibits the growth of more pathogenic bacteria. We kind of know that if we washed our hands with antibiotics every day, we may be destroying the good bacteria and giving some exotic bacteria resistant to all known antibiotics a chance to infect and kill us.

Let's use penicillin-resistant bacteria as an example. Once upon a time, this did not exist. Sure, occasionally some bacteria would get a mutation and be resistant to the effects of penicillin, but that did not give the bacteria any competitive advantage, otherwise, eventually all the bacteria would be carrying that gene. The normal bacteria have already been optimized to be able to outgrow any new mutations.

Now if you invented penicillin and started giving it to people, those bacteria would now have a big competitive advantage and take over the population. We have lots of penicillin-resistant bacteria now. If suddenly the world did not have penicillin, the historical normal bacteria would soon (50 years) regain its place as the prominent type.

Now we ingest not only antibiotics, but all kinds of chemicals not previously seen by your gut for the last six thousand years. Some are antibiotics, some are pesticides, and some are preservatives. You put preservatives in food to keep bacteria from growing. Do you think that may affect your gut bacteria?

As time goes on, most people have a different gut microbiome than people had a few hundred years ago. Is this part of our obesity, diabetes, cancer, autoimmune disease, dementia problem? Probably to some extent.

I hate to say this, but there probably is no safe level of a chemical that we previously did not in our diet. We have gotten good at measuring the parts per billion, but maybe one part per trillion will give some species a competitive advantage, and now, we have a slightly different biome. Maybe it won't make any difference, but I doubt if it will be helping us. Otherwise, we would have had that bacteria biome long ago.

The significance of the biome in disease is becoming more apparent. Many elements affect this biome, but diet must be considered to be the main components. Our diet has changed more dramatically in the last 300 years than in the previous 3000. It is not crazy to think that the modern western diet has affected our biome. It is also not crazy to think that the increased incidence in many diseases may be related to this.

It does turn out fasting affects the gut biome. It appears it may enhance bacteria richness and diversity in the biome, and it may revert to a more natural biome, one not inhibited by the overgrowth of certain species. Your biome does have a baseline. Under the influence of diet and environment, there can be an overgrowth of bacteria that normally would only be present in a trace amount. This may be part of the benefits of fasting. As you will read later, it only took five days of artificial sweeteners to demonstrate a notable metabolic change in glucose tolerance. It may only take a short time fasting to change the biome to a more favorable condition.

One of the mechanisms by which the gut biome may be causing us harm is by modifying the permeability of the gut. The cells in the intestines are designed to limit the proteins that are absorbed. Usually, amino acids can penetrate the walls to be absorbed into the body. There is a substantial immune blockade to limit foreign matter from being taken into the blood. Abnormalities in the gut biome may damage this barrier allowing immunogenic molecules to be absorbed. These may activate the immune system such that an immune reaction is generated against these molecules.

It appears that a diverse natural gut biome does tighten some of these junctions between cells and decrease systemic inflammation. Absorption of immunogenic molecules may activate the immune system to attack similar molecules that compose the normal human system.

Currently, there is interest in how the gut biome directly affects the brain and our actions. There is an extensive nerve supply through the vagus nerve to the gut, and we believe certain gut conditions may influence the brain. Specifically, does increasing the glucose in our diet affect leptin and our appetite. Previously I thought artificial sweeteners lead to an increased desire for sweets through a mechanism involving the taste buds. Now I am not so sure. Using artificial sweeteners affects the gut biome, and does this influence the brain to eat more sweets? We already know the use of these sweeteners does not lead to weight reduction, regardless of the lack of calories contained in these products.

It would take another book and research to give a decent report of the biome. Most of the study currently focuses on specific diseases. My books on Diet and Health focus on the prevention of disease based on a proper maintenance diet, not treatment for specific diseases.

I do write a little about the treatment for diabetes and obesity, which is the result of a poor diet.

Some things I am pretty sure of:

Your gut biome has a significant effect on your health and is involved in several diseases.

Abnormal permeability of the gut wall may be responsible for the increase of autoimmune disease and is related to the gut biome.

Diet and fasting affect the gut biome and can be used to induce beneficial changes in the gut biome.

Numerous modern environmental factors have adversely affected our gut biome.

Medications can adversely affect the gut biome.

What happens to the gut biome when you fast? The biome still gets nutrition from the entero-hepatic circulation (bile) and from the cells that are being continually shed by the gut.

CHAPTER 12
Fasting and Disease

I have already discussed a general metabolic benefit that can be achieved with fasting, one that has been recognized for thousands of years. Let me talk about a few specific diseases that even modern medicine has considered fasting to be a treatment.

Rheumatoid arthritis(RA) is an autoimmune disease in which the immune system attacks the synovial membranes of the joints. We do not know the cause, but everyone agrees it has something to do with environmental factors as well as genetics. Different diets have been used to show improvement, as well as fasting.

It may have a slight genetic disposition. For instance, about 1 % of the population in the US have the disease. If your parents have it, it goes up to 3-5%. If your identical twin has it, it goes up to about 15%. These numbers indicate that although genes may be slightly involved, it is probably not the cause. We are already sure environmental factors are important, and of course, your immediate family has a somewhat similar environment. The incidence of this disease varies in different parts of the world, as it does with most autoimmune diseases. Like many other diseases, once you move to western civilization from your native country, you begin getting western civilization disease, and rheumatoid arthritis is one of these.

Diet therapy has been extensively studied, as has the gut microbiome. This disease, like many other autoimmune diseases, may be based upon the biome. Later I will discuss celiac disease, and this disease is kind of a model for RA. In celiac disease, you have a somewhat genetic predisposition that is activated by exposure to the gluten molecules. This exposure is related to the gut permeability to proteins. This permeability is related to the gut biome, which is related to environmental factors. Although not the same, RA has a similar model.

Many different diets have been proposed. Generally, they are more plant-based. This may be partially due to modern medicine being opposed to meat diets. These diets tend to be based on trying to reduce the general inflammatory response in the body. As I discussed in my book *Maintenance Diet for the Modern Man,* our diet is now slanted in favor of a much higher omega 6/omega 3 fatty acid ratio then has been present through much of history. This is related to our increased ingestion of soy, and the elevated ratio in the meats finished with soy. All meat is not equal, and most of these studies do not address this issue.

In any case, our focus is the gut biome. The modern diet has changed this biome as I discussed in the previous chapter. What can we do to help this condition?

Avoiding environmental toxins that were not present for most of history will help. To do this, organic food offers some help. There is a decreased chance that these will contain trace amounts (those within FDA limits) of various herbicides and insecticides than non-organic. The FDA limits are based upon the safety of the consumer and are generally in parts per billion. It is likely the biome can be affected by parts per trillion. Of course, wash the food before eating, not necessarily to get rid of bacteria, but rather to get rid of chemicals. Increased plant intake also increases the variety of bacteria intake, which may benefit the gut biome. No matter how much you wash the plant, you cannot get rid of all the bacteria. Many recommend minimal cooking. Again, this gives us a little better variety of bacteria. Most beef, chicken, and pork products are cooked and do not contain heavy loads of bacteria.

OK, we are reducing general inflammatory factors by reducing soy and looking for grass-finished animals. We are increasing the diversity of bacterial intake, and we are trying to limit modern environmental chemicals, especially those only existing the last couple hundred years. Where does fasting fit in?

Numerous studies have shown some benefits from fasting. Unfortunately, sometimes they call a reduced-calorie diet fasting, and as we have seen, this is a different metabolic state (even a very reduced-calorie diet is not fasting). As I said in the last chapter, fasting enables a more natural gut biome to appear. Your gut biome is designed to help you survive; this means it will help you survive even if you don't have food available 24 hours a day. We can eliminate some of these less hardy bacteria. Usually, pathogenic bacteria are less hardy and can only take over the natural bacteria if we give it some type of nutritional advantage, such as a high carbohydrate diet or some chemical (medicine) to which the natural bacteria are more sensitive. Fasting can give you a gut biome reset.

Now the question is how much fasting. No one is going to do an Angus fast which probably did completely reset his gut bacteria. Studies show that although a couple of weeks of fasting helps, the inflammatory problems return a few weeks later. Fasting can only be used to help in the context of a good maintenance diet in which fasting is a part. Fasting two days a week for an extended period of time is probably enough to get a natural biome established. Of course, this must be coupled with other changes like starting the maintenance diet. I will discuss the maintenance diet in a little while.

Now is a good time to discuss Type 2 diabetes (T2DM) and a practical approach. Fasting and diet therapy can be used for RA. Let's use an example how fasting and diet can be used to treat a much more common disease.

The best approach is to prevent T2DM to start with. Therefore, I will give an example of prediabetes and how fasting is a part of this treatment.

We now diagnose prediabetes as a condition in which either your fasting blood sugar is between 100 to 125 mg/dL (it used to be higher), or your HgbA1c is between 5.7% and 6.4%. We think at this point that there is probably some insulin resistance, a condition in which it is requiring higher insulin levels to lower the blood sugar.

Say we have a fifty-year-old, somewhat overweight woman who goes to the doctor and gets a screening test that shows her HgbA1c to be 6.3%. This did not happen overnight. For the last ten years, this person has been slowly gaining weight. By weight, I mean fat. She probably knows this and probably does not want to be fat. She probably has gone through several diets, starting out like everyone else with just eating less and trying to exercise more. This is the reduced-calorie diet, probably the most failed diet, and the most often recommended diet by health professionals. When this fails, as it usually does in the long run, she started to buy diet books. Some of these diets worked if she stayed on the diet, but most of the time the weight slowly returned.

This person is normal and has common sense. She did learn something from all these diet books and probably knows excess carbs are making her fat. She also knows that as time goes on and weight goes on, she is increasing her risks for numerous illness including T2DM. At this point, despite her efforts, she is pre-diabetic.

How did this happen? I do not believe she has a knowledge deficient, in fact, she probably knows more than most about diet. Her health care provider says that the problem is a lack of willpower, but what does that mean and how can you treat it. Since we now have at least 40% of adults with T2DM, prediabetes, or obesity, is there an epidemic of lack of willpower?

Smokers obviously know that this habit is not good for them. Most alcoholics know that it is not good for them. Drug abusers know that is not good for them. They all know the ultimate treatment is to just stop. In fact, that is probably the only treatment other than giving them patches, gum, or replacement drugs. I guess we could also treat prediabetes with drugs (amphetamines), but we do not like the risk/benefit ratio.

So, the treatment is easy. Just tell them to lose weight. Health care providers could see 75 patients a day and go home early. T2DM would go away. I would not have a book to write. This is in fact what providers are telling people with prediabetes, "Just eat less".

This does not work most of the time. If someone has a heart attack, you can tell them to stop smoking, and maybe they will, even if that has not worked the previous fifty times you told them that. Same with an alcoholic who has hit bottom. Sometimes they will stop if you just tell them to. If you go to jail or almost die from drug abuse, sometimes they will stop.

I do not know why people get addicted to certain drugs, and many smart people have tried to figure this out, yet drug abuse and T2DM rates are not dropping (smoking does appear to be dropping, mainly through price control). Again, the treatment seems to be just to stop, although it may be important to understand the big picture, the treatment is unchanged.

What about our current patient? Am I saying her problem is that she is addicted to carbohydrates or eating? We would like to change this behavior while it is easier to reverse the metabolic side effects. Is this problem related to genetics or the effect of food on the brain? Is it psychological with food providing a replacement for something lacking in her life or perhaps a compensating mechanism for anxiety? Perhaps it is environmental with some element in our modern society producing this result?

In my other books, I have discussed in detail how the modern western diet has contributed to the epidemic of obesity. Its basis is the development of insulin resistance, which our current patient has. Right now, I am interested in treatment. We are going to take the patient as she is and not tell her she has been eating too much for the last twenty years. That doesn't help anyone. Now we want to treat it.

Since this is a fasting book, you can guess fasting may be a part. Not the Angus fast, but a little fasting that contributes to the overall diet. I can say that there is no doubt we are going to have to change the diet she has been on the last 25 years. At the same time, we must address the problem with the failure of all the other diets. As you remember, the main cause of failure of any diet is that the patient gets hungry. I am not talking about someone starving, but rather hunger driving the person to stop the diet. We need both a weight-loss diet that may help the hunger problem, and a maintenance diet that will prevent this problem from coming back.

If you paid any attention at the beginning of the book, you know by now that we must reduce the fat in the body, lower the carbohydrates in the diet, and try to reverse insulin resistance. We must put out the fire before we can practice prevention. Most studies show that just a 5-10% reduction in weight has a great effect on lowering the glucose level. Most of this weight loss (after initial fluid loss), is going to be fat. Lots of people can lose a little fat, but we need a lifetime diet. It took 10-20 years to get to the metabolic trouble we are in now, and it will take a while to reverse some of the changes.

I have been telling you to let 12 hours elapse after eating the last meal of the day until the first of the next day. We start this immediately. Not only will it begin to induce certain enzymes, but we limit eating to 12 hours a day. This alone lowers the number of insulin elevations which caused insulin resistance in the first place. If we changed nothing about her diet, just getting her to eat no more than three times a day would be a great start. Of course, for her, we must do more because it is too late to prevent insulin resistance. Maybe if we could have done this 25 years ago, we would have a much less chance of insulin resistance today. We are going to take her as she is.

Many of you will say we need to go straight to ketogenesis. You would be correct. Eventually, this lady will need to be on a lower carbohydrate diet. We need to get ketosis which will require a diet of

25-50 grams of carbohydrates. If she is like most people in the US, she has probably been eating about 150-250 grams of carbs a day. If you had lung cancer, you would have to take chemotherapy. Now you must go on low carbs. There are a thousand books on low carb diets. You should have no problems finding what to eat.

By now, she has probably already tried the low carb diet. If you have ketones in your urine, you should lose fat. If you are not losing fat, you are not doing the twelve hours fast daily. If you are doing that and still not losing weight, you must continue a little while longer (you should see results in at most two weeks). If you are still not losing weight, something is wrong, and I don't know what to advise. Maybe your ketone strips are not working. As a last resort, I would advise her to go on the 5:2 fast in addition to everything else. We really do not want to do this right away as we need to induce her enzymes that make fatty acids. She failed all the other diets because she became hungry. I do not want that to happen again, although I know she may have to put up with it for 2- 3 days. Even if you did not eat anything, and I guarantee you will lose weight, you are only hungry for 2-3 days.

We are on the ketogenic diet that I have been discussing. I consider the ketogenic diet to be the best fat losing diet We are trying to alleviate hunger, and if I tell you to eat whenever you are hungry (except those 12 hours), then that goes a long way toward the fear of hunger. I agree it can sometimes get boring, but too bad. We need some tough love for those 20 years you were not on a good diet.

This may be her last window of opportunity. Once you get to T2DM, even if you lose weight and your blood sugar is normal, you still have increased health risks. I am quite sure that if she did nothing this is where she would end up. She will not die immediately, and it may take years for her condition to advance, but the most likely outcome will be rising blood sugar requiring medication and eventually ending up with insulin. Along the way, her health will deteriorate, and her obesity will probably progress. There is no natural healing at this point.

If you recall, you know I am not a big fan of exercise to lose weight. It takes a lot to make any difference, and people simply cannot do that much for a lifetime. If you are running 10 miles a day, you will lose weight regardless of your diet. You will also eventually injure yourself. You will eventually have other responsibilities so that you can't take 2-3 hours out of every day to exercise. You will not have the 1-2 hours every day to recover from this exercise. Someday you may have to get a job. Recall my example of the largest loser.

If you exercise you will increase your muscles' demand for energy. If we are on a low carb diet, we are already decreasing carbs, so the insulin we have has to work a little harder to meet the demand for energy. The muscle must increase the number or functioning of the insulin receptors. I believe we are inducing the body to increase insulin receptors. Remember, the underlying pathology is insulin resistance, so it may be that exercise does reduce this resistance slightly as eventually, we get more or better receptors. The same amount of insulin does a better job. Maybe not, but at this point, I am pulling out all the stops.

I believe in this enough that for this patient I would advise a personal trainer at the YMCA, and you know how cheap I normally am. It's not that price is no object, but we are going to save this woman hundreds of thousands of dollars in medical expenses if we can prevent her from developing T2DM.

I am going to advise her to join some type of group. Maybe an exercise group at the YMCA, maybe an exercise partner, maybe Weight Watchers, maybe her neighbor. I usually do not keep track of weight, but there is a psychological advantage to her if someone is keeping track of it. It appears that seeing her health care provider helps. When we treat people for diabetes there is a direct correlation between how often they see the provider and lowering of the HgbA1c, no matter what the specific treatment. People want to please the physician, and we are going to take advantage of that. We are all in on this lady.

Finally, we are going to fast. Not the 12 hours fast; everyone is doing that every day. We are going to start with the 5:2 fast. You eat dinner on Sunday evening, then do not eat till Tuesday Morning. After you have been in ketosis for a few weeks, your body has ginned up fatty acid production. It has plenty of energy and now hunger is driven by psychology and cravings more than a demand for cell energy. If I tell someone that they can eat as much low carb food on non-fast days as they want, I find they can accept fast days.

I am going to make sure she remembers hunger is good. Ghrelin helps her brain. Fasting helps autophagy (see later this book). I am going to emphasize fluid intake as now environmental toxins in the fat coming out of her need to be diluted. Also, fluid intake helps with hunger.

Eventually, after many months, I may get her to fast two days in a row. This is not so much for physical benefit as for a psychological benefit. Once the fear of fasting (hunger) has been overcome, there is a great self-confidence boost that you can go without eating. This lady will never be able to outrun a professional athlete, but she may be able to out fast anyone on the football team.

This is an example, and you may be telling yourself that I am being a little too aggressive. This may be my only chance to save this person. I know I encourage the 30-year maintenance diet, but this lady came in with appendicitis. We need to do an appendectomy and not mess around, even if we must do it under local. Sure, it may hurt a little, but it has to be done. We could do nothing, and she might survive; but we are not.

This lady is in ketosis. How long does this go on? The ketogenic diet is temporary, and I do not advise that for a lifetime, rather I advise staying on the diet until we reach a predetermined weight. I also advise you to go out of ketosis for a day about every three weeks by eating a higher carb meal. Then return to the diet the next day. This is to maintain a more balanced endocrine system. This woman is here not just to lose weight, but to prevent the development of T2DM. She is right on the edge, and we must do what we have to do.

Probably her A1C will be going down. It may take six months to a year to get it down to normal. I usually don't like people to be on the ketogenic diet that long, but we must take it case by case. Her fasting blood sugar may go to normal. We started by assuming this patient had insulin resistance. Have we cured it?

One of the first signs of insulin resistance is a slightly abnormal glucose tolerance test(GTT). We have done millions of these tests and have a good baseline as to what is normal. Nowadays we can also test the insulin levels along with the blood sugar. If we finally get to a normal GTT, we may have reversed her insulin resistance. Now we can look to some type of low carb diet in which you are not in ketosis. This is not a normal person's maintenance diet; it is a low carb maintenance diet. I can guarantee if she goes back to her previous diet we will go back to her previous condition.

This is the point where medical providers get into arguments. Have we cured this patient or not? One side says that since every test we do on this patient is normal, then she is normal. Others would say she still has prediabetes, despite normal testing.

Of course, I say the patient is in remission. She still has 10-20 years of higher insulin exposure. She also has experienced lower than optimal autophagy activity during that time. As a result, the has accumulated more advanced glycation end products than a normal person. You will understand what I am saying later in the book. In any case, I say she is not cured. In fact, if she does not change her previous diet, she will be right back to where we started. You may ask "What difference does it make what we call it'? " The reason is because of the curse of the medical profession which is Electronic Medical Records. What is the ICD code we give her? Maybe we get paid more if we code her as a prediabetic patient instead of a normal patient?

For me, it doesn't matter since I may not be a real doctor. Whatever you do, never treat a patient in the manner I have just advised over the last few pages. You may be crazy if you do. Or maybe not, maybe I am the crazy one.

The above was a fictional example of how someone could prevent T2DM. My books are written to try to prevent some diseases, not to treat them. I want people to be on a good maintenance diet that will give you the best chance of not being this poor lady. You can use your common sense to see if any of this applies to you.

As we progressed from our teenage years and ate whatever we wanted and had a stable weight, we may have noticed a slow weight gain. I believe this is due to a combination of factors including insulin resistance and a change in the metabolic set point. We see later when we are obese how difficult it is to change this metabolic set point, and how the reduced calorie diet does not accomplish this goal. We also have seen how Angus lost a lot of weight by fasting and gained back about around 5% of this weight (Even though I do not think he went on the low carb maintenance diet). This compares to the largest loser example who gained it all back.

It appears to me that fasting may be one of the only ways to practically change the metabolic set point. Let me emphasize that I do not have any concrete evidence, but my intuition is directing me in that direction. (Intuition means arriving at a conclusion despite inadequate data) I have seen this trend in reading examples of people who have used fasting as part of their diet and, while participating in a maintenance diet, seem to be able to return just eating while hungry.

This is another reason I encourage those who were obese, lost weight, and are now on the low carb diet, to fast every now and then; if only for a day or two.

Those who were never obese and are on maintenance diet fast for a different reason. That is autophagy.

CHAPTER 13
Autophagy

If you happened to read the title of this book, you understand that at some point I must talk about autophagy. I had to talk about fasting first as this comes before autophagy as you will see.

Although I am well-read and have been hanging around the life science arena for quite a while, I am willing to admit I had not paid much attention to autophagy until about four years ago. Since then, I have been able to incorporate this amazing process into my knowledge of health and nutrition and find it difficult to even discuss these subjects without referring to this process. So, don't worry if you've never heard of it. By the end of this book, you will have a good understanding of what it is and why you want to encourage it. I am going to request that you remember what I talked about in the first couple of chapters about metabolism and fasting, especially the metabolic changes that occur in the first few days.

Before we go on, let us agree on how you pronounce this word. Auto is like a car, phagy is pronounced fay-gee. You can probably even figure out the definition as it sounds like self phagy which is self-eating. So, autophagy on the cellular level would be the cell eating itself.

On first blush, you may say that this does not sound like such a good idea, but we are going to think about it a little.

We have about 40 trillion cells in the human body. We are not counting the bacteria in the gut which may double that amount. Almost all these cells have a nucleus which contains DNA. This DNA codes for the production of a million proteins required for the cell to function (this is an estimate). These proteins make up all the little organelles in the cell, like the mitochondria, Golgi bodies, all the little enzymes and RNA, and everything else that keeps the cells going. The cell is constantly making new proteins, and occasionally secreting them as hormones.

Cells can live quite a while; some a few days whereas neurons may live 75 years or so. During this time, the cells are constantly making new proteins and getting rid of old proteins and organelles. As you can imagine, parts of the cell sometimes wear out. By that I mean the protein may become misfolded due to some chemical, it may have been made slightly incorrectly, or some cosmic ray has damaged the DNA. Remember there may be hundreds of amino acids composing a protein. If the wrong amino acid is accidentally put in the protein, it still may work, just not as well. The body is rather good at reading the DNA code, but not perfect every time.

As time goes on you can see how some of these proteins start to clutter up the cell. Even some of the organelles such as the mitochondria slowly, or sometimes rapidly, start to deteriorate. You can think of it as cell aging. If you think a little more, if the cell is aging that means I am aging. If enough cells age, then the whole body is aging, and voila, this is how we get old.

Now we can see where the self-eating comes in. We want to get rid of the worn-out parts in the cell and, in doing so, stave off premature aging and all that entails. We need to recognize what a wondrous creation is your body. It is constantly making and replacing proteins, building new parts in the cell, making these cells so that they function in an organ, coordinating the organs so they all communicate and work together. Think about it. You put something in your mouth you found on a tree, and later it appears as part of your toenail. That takes a lot of work.

We can agree now that it is a good idea to replace damaged or malfunctioning cell parts; probably the more the better. We recognize this is a fundamental component of body homeostasis, which is what needs to be done to keep the body alive. Thankfully, we do not have to think about getting autophagy going. Your body does this for you without bothering you at all. It's like digestion.

You eat a great variety of food at a meal. Your body separates the various components of the food and selectively absorbs them to be delivered to the appropriate destination. Most of the time, the absorbed contents of the gut are sent through the liver where amazing transformations of a biochemical nature take place. You do not have to think about it, but you can make it work more optimally, and you can screw it up. Same with autophagy. We can optimize it, or we can screw it up. Guess what we want to do.

Autophagy: Lysosome dependent homeostatic process in which organelles and proteins are degraded and recycled into energy.

This is the definition. Let us go over the parts. The lysosome is an organelle within the cell that contains digestive enzymes. Essentially it breaks down protein into its component amino acids. These components can then be converted into energy, or the amino acids can be used to create new proteins. Your body requires energy to function. Each cell requires energy. The body does not like to waste energy. I mean this in a metabolic manner, not in the manner of playing video games all day. It does not throw away these broken proteins but can use them as energy. It is more efficient to use amino acids that are already there instead of waiting for you to eat an amino acid, absorb it, transfer it to the cell, absorb it into the cell, and make a protein.

There are a few mechanisms the cell uses and a complicated process to identify which protein has gone wrong, but we just need to understand the process.

The cell also identifies abnormal DNA. Most of us know that cancer is somehow related to a cell gone drastically wrong. We know it has something to do with the DNA being corrupted, in other words, a mutation. The cells in the body have several mechanisms to recognize abnormal DNA being created during replication and repairing or replacing them. If a cosmic ray happens to hit the DNA while it is being replaced, the body will take care of that. Autophagy is an additional way to take care of the bad DNA floating around. Again, sounds like something we want to encourage.

Now that you may be slightly interested in autophagy, I must confess I am trying to sell you something. I am planning to convince you that autophagy is a beneficial mechanism in your body that you should be encouraging it and not messing it up. To do this you may have to make a few changes in your life. I am going to try to get you to do this for the rest of your life. This is going to be a challenge, but I think I am going to succeed if you are a common man with common sense.

CHAPTER 14
AGEs

Now another topic which, like autophagy, you may or may not have heard about; nevertheless, it is married to autophagy. I will warn you that I have written this same chapter in other of my books, and any of you who have read them (and I hope there are millions of you out there) may recognize the concept. Feel free to skip this chapter. I will not offer you a refund.

This will require a little biochemistry lingo, but I am sure by now you will be able to understand the concepts, so don't worry about it.

A little about Advanced Glycation End Products (AGEs). This sounds exotic but is rather simple. The proteins and fats in your body are always undergoing alterations with removal or attachments of different chemicals. The simplest and most common reaction is for an enzyme to attach to a molecule and enable the molecule to either add another molecule or group of molecules (building things for your cell) or take something away from the molecule (digesting molecules for energy or modifying the molecule into something else).

It takes energy to put chemicals together, and it releases energy when you take them apart. Your body can capture the energy from breaking chemical bonds and use it to make other chemical bonds. Enzymes are just molecules that enable this reaction to occur a little faster, really a lot faster so that we can move around faster than slime mold. The enzymes themselves are usually preserved so that after the reaction takes place, they can move on to make the same reaction with the same molecule elsewhere.

There are many different enzymes in your body. The rate of their reactions and the number of reactions that occur have many feedback loops such that the equilibrium of the products is delicately balanced and based on many factors. The more you investigate, the more complicated it becomes, so that in the end you must conclude it is a miracle that any life exists at all. You need to appreciate that without these enzymes, reactions would occur very slowly instead of microseconds. Sometimes without the enzymes, the reactions would not occur at all.

Most chemical reactions are facilitated by enzymes, but not all. If you cook meat, you notice that cooked meat tastes different from raw meat. Usually, we think it tastes a lot better. The proteins and fat in the meat have been changed by the application of heat. Reactions occur between sugar molecules and protein/fat molecules that result in different compounds call glycated (meaning a sugar molecule has been used to modify the molecule) end products (which means this is what is left after you turn off the heat). Advanced just means that what is left over is the result of many modifications that have occurred during the process. There are thousands of these end products than can occur, although some are more common.

We figured this out without any science thousands of years ago. You cook meat and it tastes better. We sear a roast before slow cooking because it tastes better. Searing does not "hold in the juice", but rather creates AGEs that we like to taste. The same thing occurs with bread. Everyone knows that toasted bread tastes different from untoasted bread. That brown stuff on the top is composed of AGES when the heat-activated proteins in the bread combine with the sugar in the bread and form totally different compounds that many people believe taste better. Without heat, these compounds would either never form or form in such small amounts that we don't taste them. Fat also forms compounds with sugar under the energy of heat, such as when we put butter on bread and toast it. When cooking, you usually need about 300-350 degrees Fahrenheit to get the process going. If you cook it too long, you get carbon which means you broke the AGES down too far into charcoal, which does not taste great. More cooking information can be found by looking up the Maillard reaction.

In your body, this reaction can also occur. It happens much more slowly since the temperature is so low (not 300 degrees), nonetheless, it also occurs. It ends up that the higher the sugar level, the more it occurs. Now you make toast, and you get the reaction in 4 minutes. High blood sugar and the reaction may take 20 years to get an appreciable amount present, but still the higher the sugar, the more you get. Your body is of course designed to get rid of some AGES. Even in the absence of diabetes, you will still make a few.

The sugar molecules and metabolites can link other molecules together. Remember this is a non-enzymatic process and can occur between all different parts of the molecule. It seems it often will cause crosslinking that results in stiffness of cell walls, vascular walls, throughout the skin, and even in the ocular lenses. Later I will discuss its role in the nervous system (brain). There are also AGE receptors such that when an AGE (there are many types) binds to these receptors, inflammation is induced. I have mentioned autoimmune problems several times in the book and how the incidence is increasing along with diabetes and obesity, and this may be one mechanism contributing to this phenomenon.

You have enzymes that facilitate the combining of amino acids to make proteins, and you have enzymes that degrade these proteins so you can eliminate them or make something else. When you have a sugar molecule combining with a protein in a non-enzymatic manner, you do not have an enzyme to degrade this product. Your body gives it a try and can clip off various parts of this protein and make it smaller, sometimes small enough so you can excrete it out of the urine like the other amino acids (after conversion to urea), but sometimes the protein is too big to get into the urine and it ends up somewhere else in your body. You slowly accumulate these abnormal proteins and finally get rid of them when you die. In the meantime, we call this accumulation aging.

You can see we want to minimize the accumulation of the AGEs, mainly by reducing production. This is done by decreasing the episodes of high blood sugar. Your body is designed to operate with a certain level of blood sugar. Too high and bad things start to happen. Of course, having a few thousand episodes of high blood sugar over your life is probably not that big of a deal; but having tens of thousands may cause a problem.

By now you have already figured that out and how diet can help minimize this problem. Unfortunately, if you already have lots of AGEs from many episodes of high blood sugar (diabetes), you cannot make the AGES go away just by now controlling the glucose. You can help prevent the generation of AGEs and perhaps encourage your body to eliminate a few more (autophagy), but you can't turn back the clock. The maintenance diet tries to prevent disease.

A brief note about cooking. We intentionally try to make AGEs by cooking food. The many compounds formed by cooking taste good. We then eat these AGES. The question arises, "Am I raising my AGE burden by eating cooked food?"

The answer is, probably not. Remember how protein is digested and absorbed in your body. It is broken down into amino acids. Remember one of the problems with AGEs is that we do not have the enzymes to break down these abnormal proteins. Hence, we don't absorb hardly any in our diet. If we can absorb the amino acid, that means we were able to break down the protein. This has been studied and it does not appear to be a significant source of AGEs.

The overwhelming problem resulting in the generation of AGEs is glucose, and that is where the effort should be made to limit their generation. Fortunately, this is accomplished mainly through diet, which we can control. We are not trying to eliminate glucose in the diet, as that really cannot be practically obtained, we are trying to control multiple elevations of glucose levels which we have seen can cause all kinds of problems: primarily insulin resistance.

I told you we do not normally absorb AGEs in our diet. Those of you that read the fine print about protein metabolism noted that I said proteins are normally broken down into amino acids to be absorbed, but occasionally a larger protein is absorbed. This can cause problems in and of itself as these sometimes activate the immune system. Although I do not know for sure, it's possible that some of these AGEs, especially the smaller ones, could be accidentally absorbed.

If you recall, our gut usually does not let bad things get absorbed. If your microbiome is not in good shape, it can allow bad things to get absorbed. We sometimes call this leaky gut. As we discussed, getting proteins absorbed that usually get excluded can cause problems, especially with the immune system. If you have a leaky gut, you could get AGEs in your system.

This is a book about diet, and it is something that you can control. You cannot completely control all the various chemicals in the environment and water supply. Many of these chemicals did not even exist in any significant amount in our history up to about a hundred years ago, and regardless of how careful you may be, you will still get some exposure. Your body has been designed to accommodate weird things you may eat, and your gut biome and the intestinal cells are your first line of defense. Your diet will enable these to be in as good a shape as possible.

Many of you are familiar with hemoglobin A1c. This is glycated hemoglobin (hemoglobin with sugar attached). Many of you may have had this test (HgbA1c) as a test for diabetes. This is a test that measures how much of this substance is in your blood. What we are measuring is how much of the hemoglobin has been bound, non-enzymatically, to a sugar molecule. You see, this is an AGE. Like the other AGEs, once it has been bound to hemoglobin, it stays till that hemoglobin is destroyed.

Your red blood cells last about three months, hence, the level of A1c is the average amount that has accumulated in the last three months. We can determine what level of glucose gives us what level of A1c. This can tell us your average glucose level. Of course, other AGEs that form in your body are not so easy to get rid of, but this is a good example of the more glucose, the more AGE.

We normally think of this as being glucose attached to hemoglobin, but it could also be galactose or fructose, all monosaccharides. It ends up that fructose is about seven times more likely than glucose to do this. Glucose is much more prominent in plasma, so we usually just say it is an average of the glucose level, but this is another reason to avoid overpowering your liver with rapid fructose absorption and increasing the free fructose in your blood.

The glycated hemoglobin itself can cause damage to your body via inflammation or cross-linking leading to damage and increased oxidation in blood vessels. Another way in which high glucose levels can cause direct damage to organs.

You will hear more about AGEs as you go through life as now you know what they are. They are intimately related to glucose and other sugars in your body. Although glucose is involved in most AGEs, fructose is seven times more reactive than glucose. Fortunately, the level is much lower, but high fructose corn syrup can contribute a lot. It appears that your body is designed to be able to deal with AGEs most of the time. In other words, if you keep your A1c below about 5%, you have much fewer problems. If it goes up a couple of percent, you have lots of problems. You appear to have overwhelmed your body's ability to deal with them.

How does your body deal with them? Now we go back to autophagy.

CHAPTER 15
Stimulate Autophagy

Now you can see that autophagy may be quite handy, in fact, it may be necessary for the homeostasis of your body. Your body was designed to last a long time and it would seem logical that self-repairing mechanisms are in place to assure that it does. We already know cuts heal and bones mend, but we have also commented that many diseases are increasing in modern life and, although we may be living slightly longer, we mainly just have longer times of disability.

As we think more about it, this may be the primary method by which people were able to live so long. If we think about it, many elements of the modern western diet have put pressure on your body's ability to rehabilitate itself. In my other books, I have discussed the increased and more rapid absorption of glucose. I have just discussed how elevated glucose contributes to these AGEs. Previously we discussed the gut biome and how adverse effects of diet and environment may also put a greater burden on autophagy.

Let me review it in a little more detail.

AUTOPHAGY: A lysosome dependent homeostatic process in which organelles and proteins are degraded and recycled into energy. This is the compact definition, but I need to explain the definition. This is just the lingo of biochemistry and something you will easily understand.

A lysosome is a spherical vesicle found in almost all cells. It is an organelle, meaning it is part of the living cells and can manufacture different chemicals and parts necessary for its existence. It is not just a balloon filled with chemicals. This vesicle contains many different enzymes and even acids that allow it to break down (digest) many kinds of molecules. Of course, it is surrounded by a membrane to keep it from digesting the rest of the cell and can engulf different particles or other organelles in the cell and digest them within. This organelle has its own receptors and can identify different proteins that have attached to abnormal proteins that need to be recycled and actively engulf these elements.

The process of identifying abnormal proteins, attaching proteins to identify them, transporting these abnormal proteins to the lysosomes, and transporting these to the internal part of the lysosome is complex itself.

Homeostasis is just the state of the cell living and maintaining a steady internal physical and chemical condition so that it lives. This means this process is necessary for the cell to survive.

Almost all cells of your body conduct autophagy. Your cells have many different components including enzymes, different organelles that make stuff, DNA that directs what is to be made, and is always changing. Biochemical reactions are going on all the time. You can imagine that things wear out. Sometimes the DNA is not reproduced exactly and can cause problems. Not necessarily cancer, but it can cause the proteins to not be made exactly right. They still may work, just not as well. Proteins are oxidized, bacteria enter the cell, sometimes other bad products enter the cell. The other organelles breakdown and need to be replaced. Who is doing the maintenance?

Autophagy is the process in which nonfunctioning or poorly functioning organelles, proteins, or DNA is disposed of and replaced. Abnormal elements in the cell can be identified and tagged such that the autophagy vesicle can identify and engulf these particles, including bacteria or viruses. When these abnormal particles are engulfed, we do not waste them, but they are broken down into components to be used by the cell to make other things or for energy. This process is going on all the time in the cell. You can see that this is a way for the cell to last forever. The worn-out pieces or abnormal pieces that did not meet quality control can be taken out of service and recycled. Cellular DNA has the information to manufacture everything in the cell; after all, it has already done so at least once. This sounds like a process we want to encourage.

What activates autophagy? From the sound of it, we would want more of this happening. It appears the primary activator of autophagy is intermittent metabolic stress of the cell in which more amino acids or energy is required. This makes sense, as if the cell is under stress, one of the first things we need to do is get rid of the deadwood. If the enzyme or protein or organelle is not performing optimally, get rid of it and make another. While we are at it, if we need more energy, let's get rid of the deadbeats and turn them into energy we need. This is almost the opposite of apoptosis, which is the programmed death of a cell. Autophagy is trying to get the cell to survive.

Perhaps the easiest induction of autophagy comes from exercise. If you are involved in strenuous exercise, and I don't mean just walking a little faster, you put metabolic stress of those muscle groups. You deplete the glycogen stored in the muscle, you increase lactic acid and metabolic byproducts, you decrease the oxygen, and you get short of amino acids. This is a somewhat strenuous exercise. Autophagy kicks in and you begin metabolizing poorly performing organelles for energy and eventually replacement of these with new ones. Now, this is not stressing every cell in your body, just the ones involved in the exercise. But for these cells, we are increasing their efficiency and perhaps size.

We do not need to know anything about autophagy to know that if we exercise a certain group of muscles long enough, they get stronger and more efficient.

Now I need to talk about induction for a little because I don't think you fully appreciate it.

There are millions of biochemical interactions going on in your body at every moment. These require the interaction of proteins, enzymes, substrates, and inorganic materials. The interactions cannot start with nothing and suddenly begin working. For an enzyme to function, the protein substrates must exist, and the proper chemical milieu must be present. Somewhere a DNA strand coded for a transfer RNA strand which traveled through a complex cytoplasm previously made through a complex process to a ribosome previous made through a complex process to manufacture a protein using component brought to the ribosome through a complex process which is transferred to the cell surface by proteins made through a complex process and so on.

I say this to show these interactions never go to zero. So, if we are making fatty acid out of triglyceride, there is always a little going on. Certain enzymes are induced to increase the rate, but it takes time to induce the many proteins involved to increase the output significantly. As the demand continues, the efficiency of the process improves. This could happen over years. Similarly, as the demand abates, the number of protein enzymes and precursors drops, but again this takes some time.

If you start eating a healthy diet today, it may be years to see the final effect. If you decrease carbs, your insulin level may drop slightly in days. It will take longer for your production of insulin in the pancreas to drop a little; it will take longer for the number of insulin receptors in your muscles to increase. It will take longer for your blood sugar setpoint to go down. It will take longer still for the adverse effects of elevated sugar and insulin on your brain and cardiovascular system to begin to abate. There is nothing you can do to accelerate this change.

If you induce metabolic stress in a cell, you will eventually induce the enzymes necessary for autophagy. Even if you don't exercise, you still have a little going on. If you do exercise, it still takes a while, sometimes a long time to induce the process. If you start lifting weights today, it may be years before you reach your maximum weight capacity.

Intermittent metabolic stress induces autophagy, but just in the tissue undergoing this stress. If you have a heart attack, autophagy is induced, but I would not do that on a continuing basis. Same with stroke. What we need is something that can induce autophagy in almost all the cells of the body, something we can repeat over a long time to get the autophagy working at its maximum capacity.

Most of you know what the answer is: Fasting. Fasting is intermittent metabolic stress for the entire body. Energy and amino acids stop coming in. The cells are having to hustle to keep things going. Autophagy is increasing. This does not happen immediately. Although we cannot measure autophagy directly, people smarter than I have determined the rate begins to increase after about 12 hours of fasting and reaches a maximum at about 36 hours. Now if you have been fasting regularly for years, you have induced these enzymes and the startup may be a little faster. The maximum rate may also be higher. It appears your body may have been designed to do a little fasting. Fasting may be part of the homeostasis of your body.

Since fasting stimulates autophagy, you would assume eating stops autophagy. You are right. It only takes a little bit of food to bring the autophagy rate down. It appears to be sensitive to protein such that half a meatball is enough to stop the increase. I say stop the increase because no matter what, there is always a little going on. This is one reason I do not support the only eat a little fast. In contains all the downside of a reduced-calorie diet, and does away with the increase in autophagy, one of the main benefits of fasting.

Maybe my advice for the 12 hours fast daily makes a little more sense. You may not be reaching the maximum autophagy induction, but you are slowly inducing the process. I think we recognize that for most of mankind's history we ate at sunup and sundown. Most of the time there was 12 hours fast at night. I do not know if we were designed to fast 12 hours a day, or if it's just a convenient accident to enhance autophagy. In any case, we are going to take advantage of it.

Maybe now you have a little more appreciation for the 5:2 fast. If you fast from dinner Sunday to breakfast Tuesday, we get in 36 hours and reach our maximum rate of autophagy. Do you think that if you did this every month (or maybe a few times a month) that you would be inducing the enzymes necessary for the autophagy process?

I know that most people do not require or participate in a fast of several weeks. Now if someone did that (again no starvation mode), at the end are they in better health, the same, or worse health?

Has your health care provider ever recommended you fast a little? Do you even know anyone that fasts a little? Have you ever fasted a little? We have gone from fasting being an accepted treatment or activity, to its being something weird done by the fringes of society. I'm only trying to get you to take baby steps by not eating at night, not only for autophagy, but also to avoid those multiple spikes of insulin that leads to insulin resistance. I am interested in health more than treatment. Many factors have led us to our current state in which there is an epidemic of diabetes and obesity, as well as many years of disability and poor health. Most of us want to be healthy until you die, and they want to die about age 80.

As I considered the historical state of man in relation to diet, it does not appear that starvation was common. Of course, if people starved, they did not leave records, but others did not seem to report a lot of starvation. People in civilization, that is cities, did not starve or the city would not exist. People lived where they could get food and moved if they could not.

Having said that, it did not seem to be an uncommon event that people fasted occasionally, probably mainly because they just did not have food for a day or two. This probably occurred more often in the winter as, despite the knowledge of food preservation, there may have been a few days without food. This was not a catastrophe. The upshot is that it is not crazy for me to assume that fasting the last few thousand years was much more common than it has been the last 100. I started out moaning about the increasing rates of obesity, diabetes, autoimmune disease, and cancer in the modern diet years. Is it crazy to attribute some of this to the lack of fasting in modern western civilization?

I have persisted with my definition of health: the ability to work, function, enjoy life and be content.

CHAPTER 16
Artificial Sweeteners

I would imagine that many who are reading this have used artificial sweeteners, hereafter called non-caloric artificial sweeteners (NAS), before reading this chapter. Many have probably also tried weight-loss diets and NAS may have been a part of that. Sounds like a great idea.

I am old enough that I remember when NAS became popular. Finally, we had an answer to obesity. Just eat your normal diet and replace some things (like pop) with products containing NAS. At a minimum, you should lose about a pound a month. Everyone say goodbye to obesity.

Many NAS have come along since then; the answer is always the same. Very few induce weight loss. Many studies have shown that NAS is just a poor way to lose weight. We tried changing the diet a little and using NAS or telling people to use NAS when they get a craving for sweets, or just use NAS for everything you drink except water. Nothing seemed to work, at least no better than the normal diet recommendations.

We used to explain this by saying that NAS are so sweet it desensitizes your brain and increases the desire to eat sweet things. I still think there may be some element of this involved.

Not so fast. It seems like it does not help make fasting any easier. In fact, it may increase your desire for carbs. Drink noncaloric liquids (coffee, tea, bone broth, electrolytes) but, if possible, avoid NAS.

Like I did with Angus and the monk, I am going to review a study that will make you say, "Why have I never heard of this?"

I am going to review a study that will make you say, "Why have I never heard of this?"

Most NAS pass through the gut without being metabolized by you. That is not to say that they do not affect the gut biome by changing the types of bacteria that are present. As we get better at testing the biome, we find that these sweeteners also can trigger an immune response causing inflammation. The more you look at them, the more problems we find.

Aspartame is not absorbed. It is broken down in our gut to aspartic acid and phenylalanine which are absorbed. Methanol is also formed in the gut from aspartame.

NAS reaches the gut biome, and something happens there. We already know your gut biome is modulated by diet and other conditions in your body like obesity and diabetes. This study concerns mice which means you can make almost anything happen to them. I usually do not believe you can apply everything that happens in mice to humans, but this may be an exception.

You take a bunch of mice and do glucose tolerance tests (GTT) on them. We talked about GTTs in humans earlier. You can also do them on mice, and we know what the normal values are.

Put glucose, sucrose, nothing, and three different NAS in the water for the mice for 11 weeks. The NAS was saccharin, sucralose, and aspartame. All the mice using NAS developed abnormal GTT. None of the other mice without NAS did, even those with sucrose water.

We then take the NAS that seemed to cause the most effect(saccharin) and give the mice a low carb (high fat) diet. We got the same result. A low carb did not affect the mice with no NAS in the water, and it did not prevent the mice who had NAS in the water from getting glucose intolerance.

Let us do the same thing except we give them a level of NAS which is approved by the FDA. In other words, we give the same relative amount that the FDA says is safe to give to humans. As you may have guessed, even with a low-carb diet, the same thing happened, and the NAS mice got abnormal GTTs. We may expect that a high carb diet may eventually produce an abnormal GTT, but not a low carb diet.

Now feed normal chow to a group of mice, and low carb chow to another group. Now use water on both groups. Take another two groups and do the same thing except put these groups on water with NAS. Metabolic profiles including energy expenditure are the same. Regardless of diet, mice with NAS had higher insulin levels and more glucose intolerance.

All these tests were also done using both lean and obese mice. The results were the same.

How does NAS cause this? Maybe it is the gut biome?

We take groups of mice fed normal and low carb chow and compare them with NAS fed mice with the same diets. The result is abnormal GTTs develop in the NAS mice. Now we treat everyone with an antibiotic for gram negative bacilli. After 4 weeks , the abnormal GTT in the NAS mice disappeared and all the mice were the same as far as glucose intolerance. The same thing happened when the test was repeated with a gram-positive antibiotic.

Now we highly suspect that the changes in the biome with NAS is the reason we get glucose intolerance, and if we treat everyone with antibiotics, their gut biomes become similar and perhaps even normal, and we get no GTT abnormality. Somehow the NAS has changed the biome such that a different species has been able to predominate and change the glucose tolerance. Treating with antibiotics negated the advantage the NAS treated biome had.

Why stop there? We get two groups of mice, one treated with NAS and one not previously treated with NAS. We then get some germ-free mice (no gut biome). Then we do a fecal transplantation from NAS mice to one group of germ-free mice, and a transplant from the non-NAS mice to a different group of germ-free mice. You guessed it, the NAS mice to germ-free mice gave them glucose intolerance. A transplant from normal mice gave none.

When we fed germ-free mice NAS without giving them a fecal transplant, they did not develop an abnormal GTT. Remember these germ-free did not have a gut biome to start with. If you have a gut biome and we fed the mice NAS, they got an abnormal GTT. No gut biome, no abnormal GTT.

When we tested for all kinds of bacteria in the feces of these mice, the NAS mice had an obvious different biome with overgrowth of certain species. Even using tissue culture we could take feces from normal mice, grow the bacteria in tissue culture, add NAS to one of the cultures, transplant the cultures with NAS added or the cultures without NAS added into germ-free mice, the ones who got the culture in which NAS was added got glucose intolerance. The others did not.

Finally, let's try some Humans. We take 381 non-diabetic people with an average age of 43 and look at food frequency questionnaires, especially regarding NAS consumption. We found significant positive correlations between NAS consumption and increased weight, higher fasting blood glucose, higher HgbA1c, and more glucose intolerance measured by GTTs. This was true even when adjusted for BMI.

If we compared people with the most NAS consumption with people with none, the composition of the gut biome was different in the two groups, with the members of NAS group having biomes similar to each other, and the non-NAS group having biomes similar to each other but markedly different from the NAS group. Also, this exacerbated the difference in abnormal metabolic changes.

The last test. We take seven healthy humans who did not normally consume any NAS. For a week on days 2-7, the FDA's maximum acceptable daily intake of NAS was given as three divided daily doses. After one week, 4 of the 7 developed significantly poorer glycemic responses 5-7 days after consumption of NAS(these subjects were tested daily). In other words, it took 4-7 days for those who responded to NAS to worsen their glucose response.

Even after this short test, the microbiome from the NAS responders changed from Day 1 to Day 7. The non-NAS responders had no change. If we look at day 1 biomes, even though there was no glucose intolerance on Day 1, the NSA responders as a group had a similar but different biome than the non-NAS responders. In other words, the responders' biome was predestined to develop glucose intolerance in response to NSA before the study even started.

The people who responded to NAS, even though they had not taken NAS previously, had different biomes from the people who did not respond. The biome of the NAS responders also changed during the week, while the non-NAS responders remained the same.

Finally, take the stool samples from two NAS responders and two NAS non-responders on day 1 and day 7. Then transfer them into germ-free mice. For non-NAS responders, transfer of day 1 and day 7 did not make any difference in the mice as far as glucose tolerance. For the NSA responders, transfer day 1 stool made no difference, but transfer day 7 stool caused glucose intolerance. The change in the NSA responder's biome caused glucose intolerance, even though the biome before the NSA challenge did not.

NSA changed the biome in mice, regardless of the mice's diet. This change led to glucose intolerance. Putting this changed biome into germ-free mice also led to glucose intolerance.

Giving NAS to virgin healthy people caused 4 of 7 to develop glucose intolerance. Transferring the stool of these NAS responders into mice induced glucose intolerance after Day 7, but not Day one. The NAS changed the biome after one week to one that can induce glucose intolerance.

Why did this happen? I'm pretty sure it is related to the gut biome. What did this NAS exposed gut biome do to change the GTT? Maybe the new biome caused a leaky gut such that the glucose was absorbed more rapidly. It did not change the amount of glucose in the gut. Perhaps this biome somehow affected insulin response to glucose, after all, the GLP-1 receptors are in the gut. Do NAS induced gut biomes directly affect the brain through the vagus nerve causing a craving for sweets? Whatever it is, it happened in one week.

Oddly enough, it may be that sugar-sweetened pop is better for you. I don't recommend that, but many drink carbonated drinks. You may notice an increasing number of people may be switching from diet to sugar. People have common sense. They realize that maybe this stuff made in a chemistry lab is not that good for you. They also are beginning to realize that maybe high fructose corn syrup is no good for you. That is why when you go to the store you see many labels saying, "No High Fructose Corn Syrup". I agree and will tell you more in the next chapter.

You can look up this article yourself.

Artificial sweeteners induce glucose intolerance by altering the gut microbiota, Jotham Suez, Tal Korem, et al., Nature 514, 181-18(2014)

We know that fat diets, carb diets, and protein diets all induce a change in the microbiome in humans. We know that sweeteners change the human microbiome as well as all kinds of different medications. We know that changes in the microbiome can change metabolic processes in humans related to glucose control. We know that metabolic byproducts of the bacteria of the microbiome can affect the integrity of the gut wall. We think that leaky gut may allow proteins to enter the body and induce an immune response with various and sometimes severe consequences. Is type 2 diabetes or rheumatoid arthritis a bacterial disease?

I remember how surprised everyone was when it was discovered bacteria caused ulcers and the treatment was to give people antibiotics. Is the gut the key to the treatment for much of our metabolic and autoimmune disease? Maybe.

Recent studies indicated that stevia-based sweeteners do not have an impact on the gut microbiome. Of course, stevia does have a few calories and is not an artificial ingredient. This probably means that all-natural low-calorie sweeteners do not have significant adverse effects on the biome.

CHAPTER 17
Your Brain

I will sprinkle a few diet related diseases throughout the book. Of course, we have T2DM, prediabetes, and obesity, but I did talk a little about RA and used that as a model of autoimmune disease. I am going to now sprinkle a little brain matter into the conversation.

Brain disorders of aging are now the leading causes of disability and death due to the numerous advances in the treatment of cardiovascular disease, joint replacement, and cancer. The risk factors for cardiovascular disease, type 2 diabetes, and cancer are the same as the risk factors for brain disease. These include a high carbohydrate diet, poor nutrition, and a sedentary lifestyle. The brain disorders most well studied are Parkinson's disease and Alzheimer's disease. Many animal studies have been done because it is difficult to do a brain biopsy study on humans. We cannot accept everything about these studies as applying to humans, but we can use the information to make better speculations.

Everybody now accepts there is an increased incidence of Parkinson's and Type 2 diabetes. In a large population matched study, type 2 diabetes had a 30% greater incidence of Parkinson's. Additionally, younger patients (25-44) had a four times greater incidence if they had Type 2 diabetes. If the type 2 diabetics had evidence of microvascular disease (damage to the kidney, eyes, nerves) the risk went higher.

Parkinson's disease is a progressive neurodegenerative disorder mainly occurring in the population over 65. It is caused by the degeneration of dopamine neurons in the brain and is characterized by tremor, rigidity, and slowness of movement, and dementia in the advanced stages.

Fasting induces a mild stress response in brain cells and as a result, increases the activation of some compensating mechanisms. The main one of interest is BDNP (brain derived neurotrophic factor). In mammalian animals this has been shown to increase the resistance of neurons in the brain to dysfunction and degeneration. Right now, we believe this applies to humans also.

Understand there is some treatment available to treat the symptoms of Parkinson's, but this does not prevent the advancement of the disease. It also appears as if ketone bodies (beta-hydroxybutyrate) have a cytoprotective effect on the brain. This is convenient since fasting induces both ketosis and BDNP. Think of BDNP as the growth hormone of the brain. Stress to the heart can also increase it. It appears, like many diseases, inflammation plays a part in the development of Parkinson's. Inflammation plays a part in most age-related diseases. Good thing fasting also reduces inflammation, perhaps through the action of ketone bodies.

Alzheimer's is characterized by an extracellular plague of amyloid (a protein) and intracellular neurofibrillary tangles of the protein tau. It is a relatively common progressive neurodegenerative disease affecting 1% of the population over 64 and 5% of the population over 85. In animal studies, almost the same result is present in both Parkinson's and Alzheimer's. The same mechanisms that are induced by stress produce the same protective effect.

Many of these animal studies on the effect of fasting on the treatment or prevention of brain degeneration also study the effect on aging. That is not unusual as most degenerative diseases are thought to be related to the aging process. So, if we can help prevent aging, we may be able to help degenerative diseases. Virtually all studies show that a calorie-restricted diet or intermittent fasting extends the life of various species of mammals. You will recall that autophagy may prevent aging. Remember AGEs are thought to be a cause of aging.

Hyperglycemia itself causes microvascular damage and is toxic to organs, including the brain. Hyperglycemia not only causes inflammation in the brain but also cognitive dysfunction. Although the brain does not need insulin to use glucose as an energy provider, insulin does interact with receptors in the brain and, like other tissues, can become insulin resistant with continued high levels. These receptors control numerous other pathways unrelated to energy use and high insulin may lead to neurodegeneration.

Seems to be a slam dunk. High insulin bad for brain. High glucose bad for brain. Intermittent metabolic stress good for brain. Fasting, the way to get intermittent metabolic stress, good for brain. It may be good for aging which makes it good for brain. Inflammation bad for brain. Fasting good for inflammation. Ketosis good for brain.

As I mentioned earlier, fasting has been used to increase mental acuity. The Greeks recognized this and encouraged fasting. Most religions recognize that fasting seems to provide greater religious insight. Starvation studies seem to indicate a clarity of thought and memory increases with fasting. Although I do not believe all animal studies translate in humans, fasting does seem to increase cognation, learning, and memory.

I don't know if this is an effect of ghrelin, or the switch to ketones as the main source of energy. Some believe it's the lowering of the insulin levels that contribute to this effect. As I get older, I realize we will never be able to determine the exact reason as the brain is just too complex. We are relying on observation, just like the Greeks.

We do observe there is an association between abnormal forms of amyloid proteins and tau proteins in Alzheimer's disease. Taken altogether, it does seem like autophagy may be able to remove some of these abnormal proteins, just as it does everyplace else in the body. It also seems that elevated insulin levels may increase these proteins.

The diagnosis of various dementias is also increasing in the modern era. Maybe you think this is just due to more old people, but the lifespan has barely increased compared to a few thousand years ago. I am sure the level of insulin has increased and the amount of fasting decreased has decreased compared to historical norms.

There are now many studies examining the relationship of intermittent fasting to dementia. We need to clarify our terms.

When I say fasting, I mean no caloric intake. Some of these studies consider fasting to be just a very reduced caloric intake. A very reduced caloric will result in a lower insulin level over time, as reduced calories generally also means reduced carbohydrates, but it does not increase autophagy.

Autophagy may be the main protection from dementia, but this is over a lifetime. Nobody compares people on the maintenance diet (which does include a little fasting) to those not on this diet, as we don't have many on this diet for thirty years. We can look back in history at the diets which were more like our maintenance diet than anything in the last couple hundred years; we do not see the levels of dementia we see now. Of course, it is hard to compare diagnoses from two thousand years ago to the present time, but there does not seem to be a plague of dementia in the past.

By now you know about autophagy. What do you think? Would a lifetime of encouraging autophagy reduce the risk of dementia? I know it would reduce the incidence of T2DM and obesity, but I think it would independently reduce dementia also.

CHAPTER 18
Fat Kids and Fasting

This is a slightly difficult subject as you cannot find many studies about fasting in children. There may be a few studies on starving, but we are interested in fasting. Most of us realize that fasting may not be a good idea when children are rapidly growing. It would be difficult to stop children from eating during that phase.

When kids are growing, they get hungry. You do not have to do anything. Their body directs the consumption of nutrients during a growth phase. It's like the first part of most adult's lives. They simply eat when they are hungry and stop when they are not, and their weight remains almost the same, although in children it is not the weight but the BMI that remains the same. I discussed this before as something in the modern diet causes this mechanism to go awry. What has happened is insulin resistance. Now we are on an upward spiral of BMI unless we do something.

A teenager's body tells them they are hungry, and they eat. We are not going to restrict calories in growing children. We may change the food they eat, but like the historical diet, we want them to eat when they are hungry and not eat when they are not. Even though we are not going to restrict calories in children, we still have a lot of wiggle room.

Let's agree that children are not just small adults. That is why we have the specialty of pediatrics. The continuing question in society is, when does someone become an adult? In restaurants and movie theaters we use age 12 as the dividing line. Bar mitzvah occurs at age 13. Driving starts at age 16, You can sign a contract and join the army at age 18. Of course, theoretically, you start drinking alcohol at age 21. Your full height growth may be around 23. Your brain growth may be 25. Physically you probably reach full growth at 30.

Different cultures make different decisions. Historically, the most practical was that when you were able to get pregnant or work as an adult, you were an adult.

This may be interesting, but right now I am concerned about fat kids. In all of history, children started eating at the adult table around age 3-4. They may have required a slightly different diet before then, but at the adult table they ate the same food, only less. They were eating the same as their parents.

In this present time, we are at the point that about 30% of children are overweight or obese. That may be slightly better than the 40% of adults who are overweight or obese. This makes some sense as the children are eating the same things as the adults. But like adults, the problem may be not only how much they eat, when what they eat, when they eat, and when they don't eat.

I am going to assume that about age eight the metabolic systems in the body are like adults, and they react the same way to insulin, leptin, glucagon, and fructose as adults do. If you are an obese child, you may have some elevation of your blood glucose over what would be normal for your age. Maybe you have a slightly higher insulin level than the rest of your age group. I am not certain, but I do know that like adults, you can't get obese without insulin shoveling glucose into fat cells.

At this point, we need to talk about genetics. It's easy to say that if you have fat parents, and the children are eating the same food they do, you may get fat kids. It appears more complicated than that.

A lot of studies have been done trying to find the fat gene. We know that fat parents often have fat kids, but when did this start? There did not used to be 30% fat children just like there didn't used to be 40% fat adults. Did some global mutation take place in western civilization in the last 100 years such that now these children have some kind of genetic defect?

Several genes have been uncovered that may contribute to the propensity to get fat, but there is no gene (with rare exceptions) that we can point to and say, "you will be fat". We cannot do prenatal genotyping and say this child will be fat, so we need to change this gene in the blastocyst so that it won't happen. I can be more predictive as to who will get fat by just looking at a family portrait.

Maybe you will inherit a trait such that you don't make insulin receptors as well or maybe it's the leptin receptors, or maybe your liver works a little differently or maybe your fat cells work better than most. I can say the same thing about intelligence, athletic ability, complexion, reading ability, and so on. You may need the right genes to be a professional athlete, but that does not stop you from shooting 80 on the golf course. I see this at the gym all the time. One person can work at lifting weights just as hard as another, yet some are predestined by their genes to be stronger. You may have genes that make you a little heavier, but no one (practically) has genes that make them obese. You may never be thin, but you should not be fat. Modern food has driven you and your kids to that end, but you can control this with the right diet.

Most of the time there are multiple genes involved in a complex trait. Environmental factors appear to play a much more important role. It is even more complicated now that we recognize the role of epigenetics.

Epigenetics is the study of nongenetic influences on gene expression. Essentially, we have heritable changes in the expression of certain genes, while leaving the gene itself unchanged. Some parts of the DNA may be activated or suppressed, but the DNA itself is not changed. If we changed the DNA, that would be a mutation.

The most often example used to demonstrate this involves the children born during the Dutch famine (1944-1945). These children have increased rates of obesity and coronary heart disease after maternal exposure to famine. The mother's DNA was the same; the children's DNA matched the mothers, yet the adult children manifested their DNA differently. The environment in the womb affected the expression of DNA in the adult. There are other examples of how exposure in the womb affects subsequent adults. Mothers exposed to air pollution have children with an increased risk of asthma. Epigenetic changes do not just occur in the womb but throughout the life of the adult. Identical twins may have different physical and metabolic traits as adults, regardless of the same DNA.

This makes perfect sense from your body's point of few. It is a slow process to change your DNA and the effect may not be seen for a long time. If you are nutrition deprived in the womb, it may be a good idea to change the expression of a gene to give you a better survival chance. Since the famine may be temporary, we do not want to change it permanently, only for a generation or two.

This is more reasonable than a worldwide mutation to make people fat. Now we are looking at a couple of generations instead of a thousand years. Why has obesity increased in the last 75 years? Unlike famine, adults and children have been exposed to the modern western diet, increased stress, increased sugar and high fructose corn syrup intake, increased availability for almost any food at any time, and the diminishment of abject poverty such that few people in developed countries are starving. Epigenetic changes are induced all the time and have been for the last five thousand years. What kind of changes are we inducing with our modern diet?

OK, parents get fat on their own and their children may have a propensity to get fat. What now? Many very smart people have labored to get a better understanding of this complex subject, but what do we do?

The answer always seems to be the same; eat right and exercise more. That sounds nice but why don't you just tell them to lose weight? If I wanted someone to fast, why don't I just say, "Don't eat"? I have already tried to answer this question in the Fear of Fasting chapter. This book is primarily aimed at adults, but there can be some applications to children.

Both the adults and the children at the adult table need to be on a proper maintenance diet. I will address this issue later in the book, and how this diet applies to children. One aspect of this diet, and a theme throughout the book, is the 12 hours fast after the last meal. At a certain age, the children should be expected to abide by this rule. I am pretty sure that a couple of thousand years ago your twelve-year-old was not starting up a fire at night for a snack. It is just too logical that for most of history, man did not get up in the middle of the night to start a fire and make a meal.

I am not going to give a specific age to start this in children. You must figure that own your own. But when children started eating at the adult table, they probably went along with their parents eating habits, although there probably were many exceptions for younger children.

Now the question of longer fasts, say the 5;2 fast. I don't know the answer. I do believe that the Chinese population has increased in height in the last generation. I do believe this is probably related to the increased food security in this generation such that children had plenty of food during their growth spurts. Before that time, there may have been episodes of unplanned reduced calories. I do not believe a lean teenager needs to fast longer than overnight. Around age 18 they need to start their own maintenance diet.

At the same time, if I had an obese 14 y/o, I would have to consider the risk/benefit. There is a poor outlook metabolically speaking for her life if she does not lose weight. It is quite possible, at this point in her life, to change her metabolic set point and carry that weight loss into adulthood. I have already discussed how difficult it is to change that metabolic set point as an adult and fasting appears to be the most efficient way to do this. At the same time, a child's metabolic set point may be changing all the time. MY intuition is that it is easier to change a child's set point than an adult. It may be wisest to treat this 14 y/o as an adult, after all, she weighs as much as an adult.

As I looked through the various studies on obesity in children, the answers boiled down to exercise and diet. They also advised the identification of the obese child, screening for the obese child, education of parents and child, various programs to provide exercise opportunities or proper foods, and of course numerous government programs. I don't' think eating less and exercise is the answer, it just often fails. Let me be clearer, it fails because people don't do it. They get hungry. I have now spoken often about the reduced calorie diet.

I agree there needs to be basic education on nutrition. Just like this book, the more you understand, the more apt you are to comply. But this is not the answer. Most parents do not have a knowledge deficit about what makes you fat, just like most fat adults don't. It takes convincing and, as I hope you believe now, fasting as a part of the diet, not something in addition to the diet. This is the baseline maintenance diet.

You may need to have some sort of weight loss diet (not reduced calorie), but then the 50-year diet. And let us dispense with exercise. Despite massive evidence to the contrary, we still advise exercise to get fat people to their normal weight. Diet is what loses weight. I do not know why this is always a recommendation. By now it is just a habit. Exercise can be of benefit in many ways, just not particularly for weight loss.

Who gets the most exercise? An active 15 y/o weighing 150 pounds, or a sedentary 15 y/o weighing 225? One is active; the other is carrying around 75 pounds on his back everywhere he goes. Which one do you think has the most muscle mass? You might not be able to see it well, but it's there. For the vast middle of the population, if you want to lose weight, you got to get on the right diet.

The child eats what he is given. He does not have a job. He does not go out and buy his own food; he probably doesn't steal from the neighbors, although he may at times get junk food at his friend's house. I believe it is appropriate to lay the responsibility for the child's health on the parents. I also think it is the responsibility of the parent for the parent's health. Are we going to blame the government or the medical profession for this also?

CHAPTER 19
Fasting and Thyroid

Nowadays, almost everyone knows a little something about thyroid. We know it is somehow involved in metabolism, and that is absolutely correct. After that, it gets a little confusing. Other hormones are also involved in metabolism such as insulin, growth hormone, glucagon, adrenalin, and others.

Well, maybe thyroid is just the master controller. I agree thyroid affects other hormones, but other hormones also affect thyroid. Like a lot of the information I have given you, I make it sound like we know what is happening. Really, we know what is approximately happening. If I have learned anything about hormones over the years, it is that there is an immense complexity involved in their interaction with cells in the body, with multiple feed- back loops affecting both positive and negative feedback, with your brain adding all sorts of inputs. Do you think your testosterone jumps a little seeing the appropriate picture on TV? How does that factor into hormone control?

This is the way thyroid approximately works. Most thyroid dysfunction is the result of an autoimmune process we call Hashimoto's thyroiditis. You can have either too much, too little, or maybe for a while just the right amount of thyroid. That is some disease.

Most of the thyroid in your body in in a form called T4. This is then converted to a form called T3, which is the active form that affects cellular function. Then we have the hormone that causes the release of T4 from you thyroid. This is called thyroid stimulating hormone (TSH) which tells the thyroid to do its work. This hormone is secreted by the pituitary gland which hangs down from your brain. Of course, then we have thyroid releasing hormone (TRH) which is released by the hypothalamus, a part of the brain. This tells the pituitary what to do. Then we have your brain with many inputs to determine what the hypothalamus does.

You can see that along this process there are many opportunities either to enhance or inhibit thyroid function. I am not even counting the thyroid receptors on the cells which have their own levels of control over how much thyroid is actually used by the cell. These are then affected by the induction or suppression of enzymes regulated by DNA and RNA and so on.

This complex system in your body is the same in many other systems, who then interact with each other. Your body is extremely complicated, that is why we only know approximately how it works. We have the secretion of T4 which is converted to T3 which requires insulin which, as we know, interacts with other hormones. On the surface this may make sense as if you do not have much insulin, you don't have much glucose, so we want to save energy so we won't run out.

But by now we know that if you fast, you seem to retain your energy, and if you have the reduced calorie diet, you seem to lose your energy. Even in fasting, after a while your thyroid level appears to drop a little, despite the fact you have plenty of fatty acids. As I have told others, fatigue and low energy is a psychological state. You can be so tired that you cannot take another step, then the bear shows up and you have no problems running. Your thyroid had nothing to do with it. It is quite possible the interaction of adrenalin, growth hormone, and glucagon increased your energy, despite whatever your thyroid was doing. I will not even mention testosterone and its effect on energy.

If we measure thyroid during fasting, we do see lower levels of T3. It appears this may be due to slowing the conversion of T4 to T3. We know insulin is involved in this conversion and we know insulin drops during fasting. We also know that fasting is a separate metabolic state so that there may be compensatory mechanisms at work.

As an aside, food seems to raise the level of TSH rapidly, so if you are getting a TSH test, make sure you are really fasting, or we may falsely diagnose you as hypothyroid because your TSH is up.

Let us go back to the start. Your body is designed to keep you alive under all kinds of conditions. It is also designed to self-repair. It converts food into energy with seemingly no effort or thought on your part, just like a plant naturally converts sunlight into food. You brain and body are juggling many balls at once to just maintain homeostasis. We need glucose but too much gives us too much insulin. We need insulin but too much makes us too fat. We need a little fat. but too much affects other metabolic processes. We need thyroid but too much or too little affects other hormones. We fast and get low T3; this decreases metabolism and increases lipogenesis, but that is not what we see in fasting people.

I am officially now a new age healer. We need balance in our body. It is better not to do long fasts; we only do this as a last resort. It is good to fast occasionally. It may be that it is good to feast occasionally. Ketogenesis will get you to lose weight, but it is not good all the time.

This is why I have recommended you fast, but not too long. If you want to lose fat you go on the ketogenesis diet, but every few weeks you go off a day. Even the fifty-year maintenance diet recognizes that you occasionally have feast days. We need balance and the modern western diet is not giving us this, rather a lifetime of exposure to rapid insulin spikes.

I better clear this up a little. Feasting my not be the correct description. It's more like if you are on the low carb or ketogenic diet, every three weeks you order off the normal menu in a restaurant or maybe you go to a party or eat some high carb foods. I do not mean feasting like a roman orgy or setting a record at the all-you-can-eat buffet. If you eat more than about 50 grams of carbs, you will go out of ketogenesis. This will raise you insulin level a bit and get your other hormones in better balance. After going back on you normal diet, you will be back in ketogenesis in a couple days.

After reading through this chapter, I do not know if I helped anyone with a thyroid problem. Fasting does help decrease inflammation, but if you have Hashimoto's, it may be too late to do you any good. Hypothyroid and Hyperthyroid are diseases that require treatment. I am really interested in prevention. Fasting and this book can help you, but it will not cure thyroid problems (if you really have them) Thyroid is the most prescribed drug in the US. We are probably greatly over-diagnosing hypothyroidism. If you fast and get cured of hypothyroidism, I'm not sure you really had it.

CHAPTER 20
Wrap Up

This is a book about fasting and you know more now than when you started. As you know by now, I like to take a somewhat historical perspective and religion gives us some insight.

Most religions have a little something to say about diet which gives us a good historical context as to what people were thinking about diet through recorded history. Fasting appears to be a practice followed in almost all religions and gives me some objective information about how long people fasted.

Bahia faith fasts for 19 consecutive days a year, from sunrise to sunset, no food or drink. This applies to everyone ages 15-70. Exceptions for illness, pregnancy, nursing, menstruating. This is a 12 hour fast except during the day instead of night.

Buddhist monks fast every day after the noon meal. This is a 16:8 diet every day for almost all their life. They collect food in the morning from people in the local area and are required to eat the food. Naturally, this tends to be high carb, and their T2DM is more twice that of most of the population of the country.

Catholicism defines fasting more as the limiting of food intake to one meal without meat. On some days it is just meals without meat.

Anglicanism has lots of fast days, but all this means is to abstain from a particular food or eat fewer meals. No real fasting

Eastern Orthodoxy also has lots of fast days. No real fasting

Mormons fast one day a month for 24 hours. This is usually from one evening meal to the next, so an OMAD fast. This is a total abstinence fast.

Hindu fasts are usually from sunset to sunrise and are total fasts.

Islam has probably the most well-known fasting. It occurs in the month of Ramadan, which varies throughout the years. It is a total fast from sunrise till sunset. This is obligatory in this faith with a few exceptions and has led to many clinical trials examining the changes in body chemistry during this period. This is 11-18 hours fast, depending on what part of the year it is and your location. As expected, there are really no metabolic consequences.

Judaism fasts on the Day of Atonement. Traditionally this is a total fast lasting 24 hours. There are other fast days, but they may only last the daylight hours.

Christianity does not prescribe any religious fast days.

The Bible spans all of recorded history and fasting is mentioned many times. These range from 1 day to forty days. These may have been water fasts.

From the more recent history (about the last 2500 years), there are numerous records of fasting as a medical treatment. This is in opposition to starvation, which is an involuntary deprivation of food. Hippocrates, the so-called father of medicine wrote about 2400 years ago: "To eat when you are sick is to feed your illness". There is evidence that this is true as fasting does modify your immune response.

Do not discount the accumulated wisdom of mankind and think they did not know what they were talking about. From the observation of nature, they observed animals did not eat when they were sick. They also believed fasting improved cognitive ability, a belief not only reflected in those who do fast, but also may be explained by fasting metabolism and ghrelin. Throughout history, famous men have confirmed the benefit of fasting. Benjamin Franklin, the genius of his time, said "The best of all medicines is resting and fasting."

All through the ages fasting has been considered to be beneficial. If you think fasting is bad for you, don't you think mankind would have figured that out?

From a religious and cultural viewpoint, fasting has often been seen as a sign of penance or self-denial. Whatever the reason, the point is that people have been able to fast without apparent injury from the earliest times and have done so voluntarily. They did not require any special ability, only willingness. As we have mentioned, hunger abates after a few days, and energy and a feeling of wellbeing persists. So, it may not be such a big effort of self-control and denial if after a few days you don't feel so bad. In fact, after a week it's no big deal to keep going.

The longest fast recorded was 27-year-old Angus Barbieri, and it lasted 382 days in which he consumed only vitamins, zero-calorie drinks, and electrolytes. He was in a hospital for the first couple weeks, and we have great clinical records of the effect on his metabolism throughout the fast. He lost 276 pounds. Do you think day 7 was much different than day 70? Five years later he had regained 16 pounds. I don't know what diet he went on after the fast.

Gandhi fasted 17 times. His longest was 21 days. Brides do this all the time. In the 1920s fasting became a popular treatment for almost anything. A physician in San Antonio claimed to have helped 40,000 people with water fasts lasting up to 3 months.

My point is fasting is not crazy or unheard of. Many people have fasted for extended periods of time.

It's the 1800s and you are traveling across the old west for the promised land in California. A month away from your destination, a thunderstorm scares the horses, and one of the wagons containing half of your food goes off a cliff into the river. Would you:

Have everyone eat half rations for the rest of the trip?

Full rations and fasting every other week?

Book Review:

12 hours fast is normal. Do it almost every day.

Do not be afraid of a little fasting.

Encourage Autophagy

Maybe avoid Non-caloric Artificial Sweeteners

Do not eat High Fructose Corn Syrup

Mind your gut biome.

Fasting and Autophagy for the Common Man This is a book for normal people.

Diabetes, Prediabetes, Obesity This is a book for those who have these conditions.

The Ketogenic Diet for Beginners This is a book for those who need to lose fat.

Maintenance Diet for the Modern Man This is a book for your lifetime diet and for the food engineer.

Bread in the Modern Diet The special place of bread in history and your diet.

DIET AND HEALTH All of these books in one

<h1 style="text-align:center">CHAPTER 21</h1>

28 Day Fast

I am writing this chapter to present my observations during a 28 day fast. I have reported previously on studies regarding a 40 day fast and a 385 day fast but was interested in the more practical aspects of fasting and what I would observe as someone who has written a book and numerous chapters in other books about fasting. I did not do any blood testing or really anything special, just stopped eating calories.

I cannot say everyone will experience the same symptoms as I have fasted before and followed my own recommendations for everyone to fast 12 hours from the last meal of the day to the first of the next day. I also usually stop eating Sunday night and start again Tuesday morning. Then I stop eating Tuesday night and start again Thursday morning. In other words, intermittent fasting. I have done this several years. I will admit that for special occasions I may have changed the fasting days, and rarely I may have skipped a day a week, but for more than 95% of the time this has been my routine. Hence my experience is going to be different from someone who has never fasted, and I will explain why later this chapter.

Also, despite the title, I only fasted 27 days. This was not because of any hunger or health related issue; it was simply that an unanticipated special event occurred which made me stop the fast a day early. Again, I will explain later that when you stop fasting, you do not immediately return to your regular diet. Hence, I had to stop fasting about 2 days before I was going to have a special dinner.

I still called it a 28 day fast to illustrate to you that I still believe you must enjoy life, even when you are on a lifetime maintenance diet. Eating is one of the joys in life. Not simply to satisfy hunger, but also for the pleasure obtained from sharing a meal with other people. I recognized that it was not the food I particularly missed during this fast, but rather the company of others during a mealtime. I do believe in eating correctly, and I advise you to do this almost all the time. But occasionally there are other things that are more important. That does not mean you should gorge yourself, but there are times you should be enjoying life.

Some of you recall that during the weight loss ketogenic diet, to maintain proper hormonal homeostasis I advised people to eat a normal meal about once every three weeds. By normal I meant something with a little higher carbohydrate. Usually this is enough to take you out of ketosis, but you will go right back in again after a couple days of low carbs . Fasting for a month is not the same situation as being on the ketogenic diet as you may be in ketosis for several months on the ketogenic diet. After a month of fasting in which you are in ketosis, you go back to your normal diet which means you are not in ketosis. Being in ketosis is not a normal diet, but rather a special weight loss diet. Just like therapeutic fasting for an extended period of time is something you should only have to do rarely. It is not a lifestyle. Now everyone should be doing the 12 hours fast. Many, like me , do intermittent fasting. No one should be doing frequent longer fasts. That just means you are not on the right maintenance diet.

Let me start out with hunger. As I have told you previously, this is the main reason people fail at weight loss. This is why the most common diet, that being the eat less and exercise more diet, almost always fails.

There are three main drivers of hunger. The most important is that your body makes you hungry if you are low on energy. You need energy for the cells in your body, especially your brain, to function. Your brain ultimately is what makes you hungry. The energy in your body for your cells comes from the contents of your blood. It is going to be in the form of carbohydrates, mainly glucose, or fats, mainly fatty acids and triglycerides. You must have this to live. Now your body can live off protein, but only because it converts this into sugar or fat. You need protein for other things, but not directly for energy.

You get energy from eating, and this is manifested as a rise in blood sugar. You also get energy from eating fat, but this is more difficult to measure. It is easy to measure your blood sugar levels. Your body maintains blood sugar homeostasis, and thus energy homeostasis, by secreting insulin to enhance the absorption of glucose, and to enhance the storage of this glucose by turning into fat. The pancreas secretes insulin to keep the blood sugar from getting too high and thus risk losing this valuable energy by excreting it through the kidney. Your liver also can secrete sugar by metabolizing glycogen to keep the blood sugar from getting too low If the brain thinks you don't have enough energy, it makes you hungry.

If your blood sugar starts dropping, eventually your liver and kidney start making energy by converting protein into glucose. This does not happen as rapidly as eating or using glycogen, which is the glucose stored in your liver, but it will begin to start meeting the energy demand of your body. Your fat cells also begin releasing fatty acids, which most of the cells in your body can use directly for energy without converting it into glucose, but this also is not an instant process, and your body will initially make you hungry if there are not enough fatty acids or glucose around. The liver also eventually begins making ketone bodies out of fatty acids and triglycerides (which are just three fatty acids linked by glyceride) if there is not enough glucose around. Your brain is happy to use this for energy.

The primary driver for hunger is lack of energy. If you have enough energy, you are not driving the brain to generate hunger. You can see that if you stop eating, you are supposed to get hungry.

You may recall the glucose tolerance test in which you take in a standard amount of glucose, and we then measure the glucose level over time to see how long it takes to get back to normal. This is usually 2-3 hours, so you usually do not get hungry for several hours after you eat.

Glycogen in the liver can begin releasing glucose into the blood and extend the amount of energy available for a while.

Like every other biochemical reaction involving enzymes in your body, you can induce the process of converting protein (which you have plenty) into glucose. Glucose starts dropping when you stop eating and when the insulin gets low, you speed up the new glucose making. You can also eventually speed up the release of fatty acids from your fat cells if you induce the production of fatty acids by not having a bunch of glucose in the blood all the time, which raises the insulin, which induces the fat cells to convert glucose into fat. We want to induce the fat to go in the other direction to satisfy body energy demand when glucose falls. We want to shorten the time it takes for fatty acids to replace glucose as the energy source. We also want to induce the production of ketone bodies by the liver to make the brain happy when the glucose drops, and hence get it to quit demanding energy through hunger.

If you have a history of fasting, you simply do not get as hungry as you more rapidly switch to generating fatty acids and new glucose. Everyone who stops eating will eventually get to the same place; you just get there faster and hence experience less hunger.

Another driver of hunger is ghrelin, a hormone secreted by your body which makes you hungry. This is secreted cyclically as your eating routine dictates it, such that you get hungry around the time you usually eat. This only lasts an hour or so and will go away if you just wait. This is unlike the drive to eat because you need energy which does not go away until you get more energy. After a few days of fasting, the secretion diminishes and eventually you do not get hungry at dinnertime.

Then you have the psychological drive to eat. We have all experienced the sudden appearance of hunger when we see a commercial for food items on TV. You go into a donut shop and suddenly you are hungry for a donut. Fortunately, this hunger passes after a minute or two, but it can reoccur no longer how long you have been fasting. You can be stuffed after a Thanksgiving meal, yet you still can be tempted to eat a piece of pecan pie. There is no way your body needs more energy, and the secretion of ghrelin is long gone, yet you still can get hungry. If you can just wait a couple minutes this will pass.

The goal of many who fast is to lose weight. I lost 28 pounds. The normal weight loss would be about 0.7 pounds a day or about ten pounds every two weeks. I did continue my workout schedule which includes swimming and weightlifting; hence I lost a little more than average. Usually, exercise is not a good way to lose weight. Like the advice to eat less and exercise more, it rarely is a solution. Both eating less, which diminishes energy intake, and exercising more, which increases energy usage, lead to hunger. Unless you have mobilized your fat stores to produce adequate fatty acids, you will simply remain hungry. It requires you to be in ketogenesis, that is having ketones in the urine, to assure that you have enough energy in the form of fatty acids to keep your body from demanding more. Once you have fatty acids, you are not hungry except for the psychological drive.

If you just try to eat less, you usually take in more than the 25 grams of carbohydrates, which is more than the ketogenic diet requires, and thus never get to ketosis. Therefore, you continue to have hunger, which exercise just increases as your body is not getting enough energy. This just increases the hunger drive. That is why the eat less and exercise more diet and most other diets fail. You get hungry.

You can induce your energy production to occur more rapidly. When I say induce, that really means epigenetic changes have occurred in the expression of the DNA This occurs over a long period of time in most cases. The expression of the DNA is driven by changes in the cellular environment of the cell which is primarily related to your diet. It was not difficult for me to observe that swimming during fasting did not elevate hunger, even though it usually does when I am on my normal maintenance diet, because in my normal maintenance diet I am not in ketosis. Thus, I do not have an increased amount of fatty acids floating around.

What you are doing to induce this production is increasing the biochemical infrastructure that is required to make energy in converting stored triglycerides in the fat to fatty acids which are released. It takes numerous enzymes to make this possible, and what you want to do is to increase the number or functioning of these enzymes and other processes to respond to decreased energy more rapidly. Episodes of fasting, both the 12 hours daily fast and perhaps occasional intermittent fasting is the way you do this. This does not happen overnight, but your body will eventually adapt by changing your biology.

I also paid attention to my ability to pump iron. When you stop eating your body begins to make new glucose from protein. Your brain likes to use glucose as do all the other cells in your body. The rest of your body is fine with fatty acids, but the brain needs glucose or ketone bodies. Your baseline glucose will fall when fasting to about 60% of normal, but it does not go to zero. Hence you are using up protein to make glucose, and I wondered if that was going to be reflected in the amount of weight I could lift. I have been lifting weights almost all my life and have a pretty good ideal of the maximum number of reps I can lift of a particular weight. This changes slightly based upon how much I have been working out or the health state of my body, but I am used to these adjustments. After I had been fasting for a week, I noted my capacity to lift diminish about 10%. This seems to have occurred a little too rapidly as I don't think I could have lost that much protein to affect my lift, but after two weeks it diminished to 20% of my normal lift. At the end of the fast it had stabilized to about 25%

Throughout my life there have been times when I have been unable to lift regularly either through injury or circumstances like Covid. Those who have been lifting regularly may have realized that the brain controls how much you can lift. We all have heard of feats of strength under stress or great anxiety, or other circumstances such that a woman might be able to lift a great weight that has fallen on one of her children. I used to think that it was just adrenalin allowing the muscle to function better, but now I realize the brain may be a bigger factor. Your brain protects you from injuring yourself by not allowing you to lift too much. Adrenalin may be lifting this restriction as well as increasing muscle function. I have recognized that once I have lifted a certain maximum weight, it becomes easier for me to do it again, even if I have not lifted in a while. Apparently, my brain knows I can do it without injury.

I don't think my decrease in lifting capacity was due to the minimal amount of muscle loss secondary to metabolizing protein as much as my brain limiting my weightlifting. It may be that the fasting condition affects the brain to limit your lift, more so than any minimal protein loss. I will investigate this more in a future book on diet and exercise in a couple years.

It appears to be a rule of thumb that if you stop lifting for a month, it takes two months to get back to normal Stop for six months and it takes about a year. This happened to me during the fast. In two months, I was back to where I started before the fast.

I have written other chapters on the gut biome and continue to learn about the changes which occur with diet. As others have mentioned who have undergone fasts, your stool decreases markedly in volume after about a week. Usually you would expect about 30-40% of your stool to be composed of bacteria. The rest would be related to your diet. If you stop eating, you stop passing indigestible food matter. You also diminish the amount of your dead bacteria. This makes sense as your bacteria thrive on the nutrition in the food that is not absorbed. As eating stops, you would expect the number of bacteria to decrease. In fact, why do you have any stool.

If you stop eating, does the gut biome die? The answer is no. The lining of your intestine has a rapid turnover, and your gut biome uses these dead cells for energy. You also continue to have an enterohepatic circulation of bile which your gut biome can digest and use. So, although your stool volume may markedly decrease, it does not go to zero. You still have some dead bacteria.

I previously discussed resetting your gut biome for health purposes, and one way to do this is to fast. The less hardy bacteria, which usually can only grow to prominence via a poor diet or ingestion of chemicals other than food, such as antibiotics or various insecticides, will diminish more rapidly and allow you to reset the biome. This happens rapidly, within weeks. This is one of the benefits of fasting more than a few days. There will be a book in the future on epigenetics and the gut biome.

I also noticed better sleep quality, I did not sleep more, but I also did not wake up as much. I did not dream about food or eating unless I saw a food commercial right before falling asleep. Certainly, your brain metabolism changes with the conversion of energy from glucose to ketones, and we know ketones affect brain function, but it would be difficult to quantify the effect on either dreams or sleep quality. Nevertheless, this may also be a benefit of fasting.

Finally, I was surprised that I experienced cold intolerance. This is related to a subject I have not previously discussed, that is adaptive thermogenesis. As I have mentioned in other books, most of the energy you take in is used just to keep you warm and keeping all the organs working. Only about 20-30% is used to keep you moving around and performing all the activities of daily living. That is one reason the eat less and exercise more diet does not work well. You would have to exercise a lot to make a difference, and most people have a job and cannot exercise all day.

Your brain and body are trying to stay alive. Many adaptations can and will occur to keep you functioning. You could eat a terrible diet yet stay alive. That is not to say you would be healthy, but your brain is functioning. If you begin losing weight through a low-calorie diet, your body makes adaptations such as lowering your metabolic rate. You must stay warm to stay alive. Most of the processes that occur in your body, including the functioning of enzymes, have a narrow temperature range. Imagine keeping your house at 100 degrees. Might be easy during the summer, but when there is a 70-degree difference outside it is going to require a lot more energy. If you begin eating a low-calorie diet, your body adjusts the amount of energy it uses to keep you warm. Hence you begin to feel colder. I am not talking about shivering, which may be increasing your energy requirement, but rather just decreasing the amount of energy required to keep you warm.

As you age your body also begins to slow down the metabolism in all the cells. It appears our metabolism does not begin slowing down till about age 60, and then only 0.7% a year Since our average lifespan is about 75, this does not make much difference to most of us. Still, this may also be a factor along with adaptive thermogenesis Many older people are intolerant of cold, yet most are not on a weight loss diet and in fact are overweight. Cold intolerance is still not well explained.

Regardless, there are many studies confirming that a low-calorie diet soon results in adaptive thermogenesis and lowering your energy expenditure resulting in intolerance to cold. As I have emphasized before, the fasting metabolic state is not the same as the low-calorie state and the adaptations are different. Your body does not have enough energy in a low-calorie state as you are not releasing enough fatty acids nor making enough new glucose. In fasting you have plenty of energy. In a low-calorie diet, you do not have enough. As long as you have fat stores, you do not have a starvation metabolic state in which you are relying on protein metabolism to keep you alive.

Your body does not have as good mechanisms to keep you from getting fat. Adaptive thermogenesis does not seem to elevate energy expenditure when overeating. Leptin resistance seems to develop early in obesity and is not keeping you from eating. Apparently, it is more important to your body to have energy than to be low on it, hence, it does not mind making you fat. You may not be healthy, but you have plenty of energy.

Still, I was surprised that I experienced some cold intolerance while fasting ,despite my having plenty of energy. I am an old man and there may be other mechanisms coming into play that would not have occurred had I been younger. Your body is extremely complicated, and I only have an approximation of how it works.

I must mention the post fast eating phase. Most of the complications of fasting occur during this phase. I had a special occasion, so I had to stop eating at least two days before it happened. You are not hungry when fasting, so you are not craving a large meal. The first few meals need to be low in carbohydrates. Many adjustments have been made by your body during fasting and eating carbs will cause problems such as fluid retention. Gradually go back to your normal diet and do not plan on a normal meal, or special occasion, till at least two days after you stop fasting,

I will do things differently in the future. Although it was not difficult to fast and I did not experience discomfort or hunger, other than the psychological hunger, I did not like the decrease in my weightlifting ability and having to spend two months getting back to my previous levels. I think I will confine my fasts to one week as I did not see a drop till after that time. It is also likely that on a one week fast it would only take one day to get back on a normal diet.

Remember I have spent a few years inducing epigenetic changes such that my cells more rapidly generate fatty acids and to begin making new glucose in response to decreased energy input, so I did not experience a very long interval between no energy coming in and full replacement with fatty acids. Most people are going to be hungry a few days and most are going to experience the "keto flu This a feeling of malaise when you stop eating carbs, either due to fasting or starting the ketogenic diet. Everyone eventually ends up the same place, it is just harder and takes a little longer in you have never fasted at all.

I had noted in the past a little light headedness when fasting. I attributed this to electrolyte imbalance affecting my blood volume and maybe my brain. I made an effort to drink more electrolyte replacement fluids which did seem to help a lot. Usually, I discourage drinking a lot of artificial sweeteners, but almost all the electrolyte powders contain this. I determined it was worth the risk and went ahead and drank them.

I have gradually become convinced of the importance of a normal omega 6/omega 3 fatty acid ratio. I hoped I would be able to achieve this by decreasing omega 6 and increasing omega 3, but it proved to be too difficult. Hence, although I do continue to eliminate soybean products and try to reduce other sources such as finished beef, I give up. The modern diet and modern foods have changed so much that I now do supplemental omega 3. In our history we never had to do that, but modern food and food processing has made it almost impossible to avoid more omega 6 in the diet. Remember it is the ratio, not the absolute amount that may lead to increased inflammation.

Paperback Books
Diet and Health
Diabetes, Prediabetes Obesity
Ketogenic Diet for Beginners
Fasting and Autophagy
Maintenance Diet
Bread In the Modern Diet
Epigenetics In Pregnancy
Introduction to Cell Biology and Epigenetics
Diet and Disaster: Food Shortage
Covid and Vaccines for Medical Professionals
Covid and Vaccines for the Common Man
Allulose and Other Sweeteners
Practical Sex for Older Married Couples
Sexuality in Marriage After Fifty
eBook A2 Milk
eBook Brain Disease and Fasting
eBook Tampons and Cancer
eBook Let's Rename PCOS
eBook Weight Loss for Women
eBook-Fat Kids and Fasting
eBook Lipoproteins in Diet and Health
eBook Autophagy and Ages
eBook Carbs for Food Engineers
eBook Fructose and Soy for Food Engineers
eBook Fasting and Disease
eBook Know Your Orgasm
(for advertising Know Your Organ)
eBook Know Your Masturbation
(for advertising Find Yourself)
eBook Know Your Clitoris
(for advertising Know Yourself)

eBook Artificial Sweeteners and the Gut Biome
eBook 28 Day Fast
eBook Dementia in Women
eBook Fat and Protein for Food Engineers
eBook The Food Engineer
eBook Flour Treatment
eBook Bread Gluten and Sensitivity
eBook Introduction to Stem Cell
(Regenerative Cell) Treatment
eBook Prolonged Fasting